New Concepts in
Surgical Pathology of the Skin

Wiley Series in
SURGICAL PATHOLOGY

Editor
William Hartmann, M.D.

Associate Editors
Saul Kay, M.D.
Richard J. Reed, M.D.

NEW CONCEPTS IN SURGICAL PATHOLOGY OF THE SKIN
Richard J. Reed, M.D.

New Concepts in Surgical Pathology of the Skin

RICHARD J. REED, M.D.
Department of Pathology
Tulane University School of Medicine
New Orleans, Louisiana

A Wiley Biomedical Publication

JOHN WILEY & SONS

New York • London • Sydney • Toronto

Library of Congress Cataloging in Publication Data:

Reed, Richard Jay, 1928-
  New concepts in surgical pathology of the skin.

  (Wiley series in surgical pathology) (A Wiley bio-
medical publication)
  Bibliography: p. 149
  Includes index.
  1. Skin—Diseases. 2. Skin—Diseases—Diagnosis.
3. Pathology, Surgical. I. Title. [DNLM: 1. Skin—
Pathology. 2. Pathology, Surgical. WR105 R325n]
RL95.R43   616.5'07   75-45029
ISBN 0-471-71332-5

Printed in the United States of America

10 9 8 7 6 5 4 3 2 1

Series Preface

Surgical pathology has been through a revolution! Although conceived by surgeons (one of many areas that can be ascribed to the genius of William S. Halstead), by the participation and leadership of pathologists, it has evolved from a subdivision of surgery to become a discipline of its own. Like all disciplines, its tools need definition. Of its many tools, the basic one is the approach to a specimen. This requires an understanding of tissue handling and is addressed to the solution of at least two questions: (1) What and where is the lesion for which surgery was performed? and (2) What is the best way to demonstrate this lesion on a slide? These questions are basic to our profession. The approach to their answers is not only the fundamental skill of a surgical pathologist, but will, in fact, determine how well the surgical pathologist discharges his responsibilities to his colleagues, his trainees, himself, and his profession.

The concern of the surgical pathologist for diagnostic and experimental endeavors is documented in the literature. We have excelled in these endeavors. We are better equipped than our professional forefathers, but may have faltered in the use of our equipment. This series was conceived to improve our "bench" job and to make this basic approach available to trainees and practitioners.

The why's and how's of specimen handling in surgical pathology are our primary concern. Experts in a given anatomic area will address specimen handling and, having done so, will have the opportunity to discourse on a subject or subjects in their area of expertise and interest.

It is our intent that these volumes fill a void that has existed in surgical pathology literature since Joseph Colt Bloodgood, the first American surgical pathologist. We do not intend them to become compendia of diagnostic criteria. Our success will be measured by how completely we answer the two basic questions. The usefulness of our undertaking will be measured by the physicians, surgeons, and pathologists in practice and training. If this is a successful and useful series, they will know, and the patients they serve will benefit.

WILLIAM HARTMANN, M.D.
SAUL KAY, M.D.
RICHARD J. REED, M.D.

Contents

Contents

New Concepts in
Surgical Pathology of the Skin

Chapter 1

Introduction

Surgical pathology was devised as a peculiar adaptation of techniques in pathology to the solution of surgical problems. It was evolved by surgeons, but later adopted by pathologists. Its history has been one of servitude. Until recently, it has been relegated to the role of stepchild. In the academic environment, it assumed the characteristics of a Cinderella whose needs were subservient to those of research. At this time, the academic disciples of pathology have turned a smiling face to their "Cinderella."

Surgical pathology has also had to share favors with clinical pathology. In a manner somewhat similar to the stepchild approach of the academicians, the hospital-based pathologist has favored the monetarily fruitful specialty of clinical pathology. The random section approach to a surgical specimen, which is used by many hospital-based pathologists, is reflected in a pathology report that is of little or no use to the surgeon. The surgeon's respect for the pathologist mirrors the latter's respect for a surgical specimen.

It is the duty of the surgical pathologist to provide the surgeon with prognostically significant information from a study of surgical material. The surgical pathologist records the gross characteristics of the material provided by the surgeon. If an immediate therapeutic decision is pending, he may prepare and interpret a frozen section of a representative portion of tissue. Routinely he sections the surgical specimen in a manner that will best demonstrate the nature of the disease process. Histologic sections are prepared, studied and interpreted. The interpretations are recorded and submitted to the surgeon to guide him in the diagnosis and treatment of disease.

The surgical pathologist functions as a consultant. His prime function is the interpretation of surgical material. He may make recommendations based upon his interpretation, but he does not dictate treatment. Occasionally his interpretations may provoke questions as to the appropriateness of surgical decisions or procedures. The answers to these questions are not his responsibility. Such questions are properly referred to a review board of surgical peers.

The surgical pathologist is skilled in the interpretation of gross specimens. His manipulations and dissections are based on knowledge of the anatomy, the vascular supply; and the lymphatic drainage of the area.

He supplements this information with a knowledge of the physical characteristics of diseases that commonly involve the area.

Many subspecialties of pathology have evolved under the direction of clinicians. The preparation and interpretation of biopsy specimens from the skin, liver, kidneys, and skeletal muscles all pose similar problems. They require special techniques and a familiarity with the terminology of clinical subspecialties. It has generally proved to be the path of least resistance to ignore these special requirements. As a consequence, these special fields often have functioned better under the direction of clinicians. Each inroad by clinicians into anatomic pathology is an admission by pathologists that they are too concerned with business to practice medicine. Many pathologists are primarily concerned with the monetarily fruitful business of the clinical laboratory and have failed to shoulder a responsibility for newer techniques in anatomic pathology.

A competent microscopist is not simply a storage site for microscopic verbiage. It is not enough to be able to recite by rote the microscopic findings once the clinical diagnosis is established. The ability to offer clinical differential diagnoses from the interpretation of microscopic findings is the mark of the mature diagnostic pathologist. In addition, he may record data that are prognostically significant or offer suggestions for pertinent clinical tests. The ability to recognize cytologic and histologic features is simply a beginning. The ability to integrate microscopic findings into a meaningful interpretation is the distinguishing characteristc of a pathologist and is the art of pathology.

Dermatology as a clinical specialty is an extension of gross pathology. It is a visual art whose practitioners depend almost entirely on visual images to diagnose and categorize disease. Dermatologic diagnoses are based on the recognition of such basic reaction patterns as erythema, edema, vesiculation, and necrosis. Additional diagnostic qualifications depend on the duration of the process, the distribution of lesions, and the presence or absence of systemic symptomatology. Once the preceding parameters have been noted, the final classification of the disease may depend on a relatively minor distinguishing detail. Often the process is then categorized by giving it the name of the physician who first defined the syndrome. The result of this empirical approach has been a bewildering terminology that represents a terrible burden for the neophyte in dermatology. In spite of these handicaps, dermatology is a satisfying specialty. It is possible to develop a diagnostic proficiency that is rarely attained in other clinical specialties.

Dermatopathology has evolved as an ancillary subspecialty of dermatology. The major thrust in its development has been the characterization of clinical syndromes by their morphologic patterns rather than their histogenesis. The neophyte in dermatopathology has been taught the clinical syndromes and has had to memorize a collection of verbiage that characterizes the histologic changes for each syndrome. With this approach, it is not surprising that there has been relatively little interest in dermatopathology by pathologists.

It is possible to approach dermatopathology as a study in histogenesis. The reaction patterns of the skin are limited. Once the histologic pattern is characterized it is usually possible to relate the pattern to one or more clinical syndromes. One of the satisfying aspects of dermatopathology is the close cooperation that is possible between clinician and pathologist. The clinician can usually supply the limits of the possible clinical syndromes.

The impact of histogenetic concepts on dermatologic terminology is just beginning to be felt. As a striking example we might consider the following clinical syndromes: bullous ichthyosiform erythroderma, ichthyosis hystrix, systematized epithelial nevus, nevus unius lateris, hard nevus of Unna, and palmar and plantar erythroderma. In each of these conditions, a histologic pattern characterized by peculiar edematous and dyskeratotic changes may be present in the stratum malpighii. This histologic pattern, which has been characterized as epidermolytic hyperkeratosis, is easily grasped by the neophyte pathologist. Once grasped, it may be correlated with the information supplied by the clinician to define a clinical syndrome.

The future of dermatopathology is somewhat uncertain. Dermatopathology has seldom been fully accepted as the responsibility of pathologists or pathology training programs. For the most part, it has remained more closely allied to the discipline of dermatology. By political design, its future will apparently be determined by clinicians, rather than by pathologists. Hopefully, it will fare better than other subspecialties of pathology, that, by default, have remained the responsibilities of clinical services.

Chapter 2
Ethics and Deportment

THE CLINICIAN AND HIS PROBLEMS

It is difficult to translate the pathologist's interpretations of a surgical specimen into a doctor–patient relationship. The examination of material that is submitted to a pathologist is initiated under the direction of a clinician. The character and purpose of the examination are generally indicated on the request form supplied by the clinician. The pathologist's written interpretation of a test is in turn directed to the requesting clinician. The pathology report is a consultation between physicians. As a result of this consultation, the clinician may request additional tests or initiate treatment. The clinician has the responsibility of translating the information supplied by the pathologist into meaningful actions for the patient. He serves as an intermediary between the patient and the pathologist. Logically, the expenses for the clinician's consultation with the pathologist should be the responsibility of the clinician rather than the patient. Ethically, this arrangement has too many weaknesses to be a recognized or accepted practice.

With few exceptions, the written report of the pathologist is a commission. Extrapolations from this written commission by the clinician must be limited in scope. It is the responsibility of the pathologist to commit to his report all positive and negative findings. The clinician does not have the prerogative of supplementing the pathologist's report with his own interpolations into the written commission. An incomplete or inadequate report by the pathologist tends to encourage the clinician to interpret the omissions as having an importance equal to, or greater than, that of the commissions. A detailed microscopic report and an equivocal final diagnosis are an open invitation to speculation by the clinician. Under such circumstances, a common histologic finding, such as liquefaction degeneration at the dermoepidermal junction, may be equated in the mind of a clinician with the diagnosis of lupus erythematosus. The microscopic report details the reasoning of the pathologist in arriving at a diagnosis. It is a statement of positive and negative findings. It has unquestioned medicolegal significance. An interpretation by the clinician of the written description of microscopic findings that contradicts or is at variance with the written commission (final diagnosis) of the pathologist is indefensible. Clinicians who violate

4

this premise should be denied the benefit of a detailed microscopic description. They are jeopardizing the value of the pathologist's report.

The commission of the pathologist is entrusted to the clinician, who has the power to act in behalf of his patient. It is not a dictum. The clinician has the responsibility of integrating all the findings (historical, physical, and laboratory) interpreting them, and prescribing appropriate treatment. The commissions of the pathologist, particularly those relating to anatomic pathology, are often deciding factors in the clinician's interpretation. They may contain more than merely a final diagnosis. For rare or unusual lesions the pathologist, on the basis of his knowledge of similar processes, may elect to provide a statement regarding behavior and prognosis. The pathologist seldom, if ever, has available all of the factors that influence the clinician's interpretations. Therapeutic recommendations by the pathologist should always be general statements. They should not be offered as specific dicta. With an adequate commission by the pathologist, an error in a therapeutic decision by the clinician should not indict the pathologist as guilty by association. If dicta regarding therapy are offered by the pathologist, but prove in their execution to be in error, then the pathologist shares the guilt. The guilt does not extend to correct therapeutic decisions that are marred by technical errors.

The philosophy of the frozen section is pertinent to a discussion of the clinician and his problems. The frozen section is a consultation between physicians. It requires an authorization from the clinician in the form of a written request that also documents significant findings. Some clinicians look upon the frozen section as a contest requiring little or no cooperation with the pathologist. A few are so perverted that they may offer misleading clinical information. The pathologist must judge whether the gross specimen and the recorded clinical data warrant the preparation of a frozen section. If they are judged to be inadequate, the request by the clinician for a frozen section may be denied. A failure to exercise this prerogative may find the pathologist compromised if medicolegal problems arise.

In many hospitals the responsibility for the initial interpretation of a frozen section falls upon a resident, who is usually capable of handling most of the problems. However, it is doubtful if a final decision to await permanent sections (no frozen section diagnosis) should be made by anyone other than the surgical pathologist.

At the present time medical ethics are in a confused state. At one time, fee-splitting was considered a serious breech of ethics. Direct billing of the patient by the pathologist for services rendered is largely an outgrowth of efforts to combat fee-splitting. With the advent of automation and the influx of funds from insurance programs, many of our time-honored standards of ethics have disappeared. There is currently a trend in several of the medical specialties for the clinician to usurp the role and the prerogatives of the pathologist. When surgical pathology was evolving as a specialty, it was a common practice for the clinician to function as a pathologist and to dissect, section, and interpret the products of his surgical endeavors. Histologic diagnoses, such as "chronic appendicitis," were common and offered justification for a number of questionable surgical procedures. The way was open for the incompetent surgeon to cover a variety of mistakes under a blanket of vague histologic diagnoses. We are faced with somewhat similar problems at present. The pathologist's hesitancy in accepting responsibility for specialized techniques, such as "thick" sections and immunopathology, has encouraged clinicians to evolve into pseudopathologists with limited, specialized skills. In the special realm of dermatopathology, there are serious objections to the clinician who also functions as his own pathologist. His incidence of errors in clinical diagnosis is likely to be remarkably low. If the clinician wishes to practice as a pathologist, he should be obliged to restrict such endeavors to material submitted by clinicians other than himself. Clearly, the pathologist should be a disinterested third party.

The competition offered anatomic pathologists by lay laboratories has made it easier for some clinicians to function as pathologists. It is possible to submit a biopsy specimen to certain lay laboratories and to obtain a satisfactory microscopic section for a reasonable fee. Unfortunately some pathologists have confused business with the practice of pathology and have offered clinicians a similar service. This practice represents a form of fee-splitting. It is not at all clear that clinicians who avail themselves of this type of service act in the best interest of the patient. Does the patient always know that his biopsy has been interpreted by the clinician? What is the clinician's charge for his histologic interpretations?

Among the many peculiarities of clinicians is a possessiveness in regard to their operative specimens. Evidence of this quirk is a disregard for hospital rules pertaining to the delivery of intact operative specimens to the pathology laboratory. Portions of the specimen may be removed from the hospital and delivered to a research laboratory or to a favored pathologist. This interference with hospital procedures may complicate the interpretation of the specimen and eventually may compromise the care of the patient. The diagnostically significant portion of the specimen may be the portion that was removed from the hospital by the surgeon. Often this violation of hospital rules may be additionally complicated by conflicting or differing interpretations by the hospital-based pathologist and by the surgeon's favorite. The guilty surgeon's reaction to this dilemma often is righteous indignation. Referral of the problem to the hospital tissue committee is the proper solution for the surgeon's indignation. A somewhat similar breed is the clinician who takes multiple biopsies, submits each one to a different pathologist, and then confronts one or more of the involved pathologists with the conflicting reports.

THE PATHOLOGIST AND CONSULTATIONS

Every pathologist has been faced with the problem of the clinician who, slide in hand, wants an immediate consultation. If the pathologist obliges, but offers a diagnosis which differs from that of the pathologist whose laboratory prepared the slide, the surgeon is vindicated in his search for the truth. The surgeon's usual reaction to this controversy is that the first pathologist was in error and should be so informed. This comedy of errors may be avoided if proper procedures for consultations are followed. Consultations between pathologists do not require the clinician as an intermediary. If a consultation between pathologists is desired by a clinician, the material should be forwarded by the pathologist to the consultant. The consultant should be an authority who satisfies both the clinician and the referring pathologist. The consultant should direct his written opinion to the referring pathologist.

The ethics of a consultation are not defined. They border on mores that have been handed down from one generation to the next, but seldom, if ever, committed to writing. Consultations may be requested on a regular basis or may be infrequent or one-time occurrences. They may be informal requests for an opinion, or an informal sharing of interesting material. Formal requests may be a search for prestige in which a definitive diagnosis is confirmed by an authority, or they may represent a plea for help on the diagnosis, prognosis, and treatment of a problem case. They may occasionally be part of a contest in which representative sections of a problem lesion are submitted to two or more authorities with the anticipation that controversies will evolve. Finally, a clinician may request additional consultations. The clinician's rationale for such requests may be an expression of conflicts between clinical patterns and histologic diagnoses or of personality conflicts between the clinician and the pathologist. They may reflect the "Mayo Clinic Syndrome" in which only one authoritative source is recognized.

For medicolegal purposes, the informal verbal consultation is practically worthless. The recipient of such a service must also recognize that a written report invariably represents a greater expenditure of mental effort by his consultant. During the preparation of a written report the consultant is allowed time to reflect upon subtle histologic changes and to return to problem areas several times for significant clues. Finally, his signature over a written diagnosis is a documentation of the thought and effort he has expended.

Formal requests for a consultation on material that is submitted with a definitive diagnosis are not particularly stimulating for a consultant. In such cases, the submitting pathologist is impressed with the prestige that is derived from a confirmatory written report by an authority. When faced with such a problem, the consultant occasionally may offer a significantly different diagnosis, but in general the challenge of the difficult lesion is lacking.

A formal request for help on a problem lesion by a troubled pathologist offers the greatest challenge to a consultant. Some lesions present problems that exceed the capabilities of the consultant. Some of these problems may be related to the way the specimen was originally sectioned and processed. Occasionally, the consultant may request additional material. In some of these problem cases, the additional material may provide significant clues to histologic or biologic problems. For occasional lesions the consultant must admit his inadequacies, but, if possible, should direct the material to a consultant with appropriate expertise. For some difficult lesions the consultant may be able to offer significant histologic interpretations of patterns of growth, mitotic rate, and biologic potential in the absence of a definitive diagnosis.

The pathologist who simultaneously submits material to two or more consultants should be prepared to reap the whirlwind. If they are informed of the contest at the time they receive the histologic preparations, the consultants may agree to participate. If they are uniformed contestants, they may become extremely agitated when faced with conflicting diagnoses.

The clinician who requests a consultation because a pathologist has rendered an astute diagnosis on an unusual lesion will precipitate a reaction of some sort from the pathologist. When the clinical picture does not correlate with the histologic diagnosis, such a request may be reasonable but irritating. At the other extreme the clinician, who has attained a degree of snobbery that reflects the "excellence" of his training, may assume that astute diagnoses issue only from the center where he was trained and may request that all unusual material be forwarded to that center for review and confirmation of the diagnosis.

Finally, we are faced with the problem of patients who are referred to specialized treatment centers. The pathology staff in these centers need not reflect the same degree of competence as that of the referral group. Verbal reports may be given to patients for transmittal to the referral group. These verbal reports are often confusing and contradictory. The patient may report that the lesion was benign but may show the stigmata of radical surgery. Several months later, a corrected report may issue from the treatment center. These treatment centers are faced with problems that require expertise and extreme care in public relations. If conflicts arise between the diagnosis from the pathology group in the treatment center and that of the referral group, it is the responsibility of the group in the treatment center to share their opinions and material with the referral group promptly.

If consultations are submitted on a regular basis, the referring pathologist should work out financial arrangements with the consultant. If consultations are only occasionally submitted, the referring pathologist should expect a bill from the consultant for services rendered. If a bill is not submitted in a reasonable period, the pathologist should contact the consultant and establish the latter's fee for a consultation. Although the case may appear to the referring pathologist to have intrinsic value for the consultant, the latter is obliged to spend his time and that of his secretary in preparing a written report.

The pathologist often receives requests from clinicians for the loan of histologic preparations. Preferably these requests should be answered by a query to the clinician for the address of a pathologist who is readily available and responsive to the needs of the clinician and the referring pathologist. By political design or by necessity some clinicians may also function as pathologists. From their review of histologic sections they may correlate their histologic and clinical findings to formulate a diagnosis. They are strongly influenced by clinical findings and tend to interpolate their clinical impressions into their histologic interpretations. Their histologic interpretations may be at variance with or may contradict those of the pathologist who furnished the histologic sections. As a matter of courtesy, the clinician should furnish the pathologist a copy of a pathology report based upon the clinician's interpretations of the pathologist's histologic preparations. Medicolegal implications necessitate such a report. If the clinician ignores these responsibilities, the pathologist should communicate the deficiencies to the negligent clinician. Subsequent requests of a similar nature do not bind the pathologist. The burden becomes that of the clinician to furnish the name of a pathologist (consultant) who satisfies the needs of the clinician and the referring pathologist.

Chapter 3

General Guidelines for a Dermatopathology Laboratory

IDENTIFICATION OF SPECIMENS FOR MAILING

The proper identification of specimens, particularly multiple biopsy specimens, is the responsibility of the clinician. Often multiple specimens are included in a single bottle of formalin. Seemingly insignificant lesions, such as cellular nevi, may occasionally prove on histologic examination to be life-threatening processes that require identification of site of origin. The information supplied by the clinician should include site of biopsy, duration, and pertinent historical and physical findings. If multiple specimens are submitted from one patient, they should be properly identified on each of the bottles of formalin and on the pathology request forms. This is best done by identifying the site with an appropriate letter or number on both the request form and the corresponding specimen container. It is also an aid to indicate the total number of separate specimens on each bottle (i.e., if there are three separate specimens, then each bottle is identified with a specific number and a total number as 1 of 3, 2 of 3, and 3 of 3).

If specimens must be mailed to the pathologist, it is the clinician's responsibility to identify each specimen bottle properly. Each formalin container should be labeled with the address of the laboratory in addition to the identifying data supplied on the cardboard mailing container. Since the lid of the mailing container is often detached and lost in the mail, and the formalin container may separate from the paper container, each of these containers needs identifying data.

EXAMINATION OF GROSS SPECIMENS

The purpose of the gross examination of a surgical specimen includes one or more of the following points.

1. Documentation of physical characteristics.
2. Evaluation of patterns of growth (if neoplastic).
3. Selection of areas to be submitted for microscopic examination.
4. Proper labeling of sections submitted for microscopic examination to facilitate their identification and to permit correlation of microscopic features with the gross appearance of a lesion.

Unfortunately the gross examination of surgical specimens is often presented to a resident as an onerous duty. This attitude may persist after completion of training. An appreciation for and feeling for gross pathology are difficult to develop, but once obtained permit the practicing pathologist to fulfill his duties with increased confidence and pleasure. If would be a mistake for this book to merely describe various routine techniques to be used in the preparation of surgical specimens. The mechanics of the preparation of surgical specimens depends, in part, on the facilities available for special techniques. The purpose of this book is to record some of our experiences and mistakes in the hope that they will benefit others.

The examination of a gross specimen and the selection of areas to be submitted for microscopic examination should facilitate the diagnosis of lesions being studied, and, if possible, should provide information about the prognosis of the lesion. The manipulation and description of the specimen at the cutting board cannot be reduced to stereotyped procedures. Routine stereotyped procedures for processing and describing specimens may become ritualized, so that the importance of the procedure in the mind of a pathologist may overshadow that of the specimen itself. Each specimen is unique and presents special problems that may be obscured or not appreciated if the performance of these procedures becomes stereotyped. If a specimen has been improperly handled, either through ignorance or through carelessness, it is seldom possible to return to the wet gross and obtain the same degree of information that would have been available if the specimen had been properly handled initially. Microsections of a difficult borderline lesion that are technically unsatisfactory because the specimen was not properly prepared prior to fixation are inexcusable. Specimens that have remained in the fresh state in a refrigerator over the weekend for the convenience of the pathologist seldom yield sections of a comparable quality to those produced by proper fixation within a few hours after surgery.

The proper manipulation of a surgical specimen and the selection of adequate blocks for microscopic examination depend on a knowledge of the anatomy of the organ and of the behavior and spread of disease within the organ. With the exception of rare and unusual diseases most of the problems in surgical pathology can be recognized and diagnosed with some degree of confidence at the cutting board. For neoplastic diseases it is usually possible to make a distinction between sarcomas and carcinomas. For lesions that can be diagnosed on the basis of their gross characteristics, it should be possible to predict the routes of spread. Sections should be taken to document the presence or absence of a lesion along these avenues. Often it is possible to anticipate the need for special techniques in processing.

The description of the gross appearance of a lesion is related to the scientific ideal that our duty as pathologists is to document and study human disease. At the practical level, the documentation of the gross appearance of a specimen has medicolegal significance that outweighs the scientific ideal. If the description of the specimen is insufficient or inadequate to allow its subsequent identification, the liability falls on the pathologist for cases in which there is a mix-up involving two or more specimens. The description of a specimen should adequately document the organ if it is identifiable, the nature of the specimen when received in the laboratory, and its size, contour, color, and other distinguishing features.

Chapter 4

Documentation of Pathology

MATERIALS

The space provided for the gross examination of a surgical specimen is usually small and cramped. It is somewhat disturbing to walk into a modern, well-lit laboratory and to find the bench for surgical pathology crowded into an inaccessible, poorly lit corner. The thought that goes into the design and construction of most work areas for the preparation of gross specimens is probably a reflection of the low esteem in which many pathologists hold this level of their art. The rapid acceptance of computerized standard descriptions of routine surgical specimens will undoubtedly hasten a decline in the ability to diagnose disease from the examination of a gross specimen.

The area provided for the cutting board should be well lit and well ventilated. It should have a table that is sufficiently long to permit the examination of large specimens, such as an amputated leg. Space should also be available for formalin-filled trays, which are required for the overnight fixation of surgical specimens. The table top should be at a comfortable height from the floor. There is some advantage in having a table of sufficient height to permit easy manipulation of surgical specimens while standing. It is then a simple matter to adjust a stool to a comfortable height for working at the same level while sitting. The surface of the cutting board should be sufficiently coarse to allow some resistance to movement of the specimen over its surface. It is difficult to improve upon the resilience of a cork board, although the porosity of a cork surface presents something of a problem when handling fragmented specimens. Wax also provides a satisfactory cutting surface. For small specimens, plates of dental wax are useful and may be discarded when no longer suitable as a cutting surface. For large specimens, a wooden tray filled with paraffin provides an adequate surface that is readily resurfaced by the addition of fresh melted paraffin.

Instruments should include a malleable probe, a pair of heavy scissors, such as Mayo surgical scissors, a pair of small scissors with sharpened points for delicate dissections, a medium pair of toothed forceps, a medium pair of smooth forceps, a pair of small smooth forceps, a scalpel handle, disposable blades, a rigid general purpose knife (4 to 6 in. long), and pins for attaching specimens to a cork, wooden, or paraffin surface. Additional instruments for special procedures include a Copen saw, a vise, and a bandsaw. Bandsaws designed for use in butcher shops are preferable to those designed for use by carpenters. A bandsaw is indispensable for the examination of large bones. Sections from hard substances, such as bone, which are to be submitted for microsectioning, are best obtained by use of a hand saw. Power saws, particularly those of the oscillating type, develop considerable local heat and produce a large amount of bone dust. The bone dust impregnates the marrow spaces and obscures the histology.

DESCRIPTION OF GROSS SPECIMEN

The procedure to be followed in processing a specimen of skin is determined by the configuration and dimensions of the specimen. These characteristics depend on the type of surgical procedure that produced the specimen. The initial description of a gross specimen should, if possible, identify the organ and the condition in which the specimen is received, whether in a fresh state or in a fixative. If the specimen has been received in a fixative, the nature of the fixative should be identified. Occasionally specimens are mistakenly placed in solutions other than routine fixatives. If a fixative other than formalin has been used, the nature of the fixative should be noted and special procedures instituted for proper processing of the specimen. Occasionally specimens are received in water. The use of an improper fixative becomes evident after examination of microscopic sections, but it is a comfort to the pathologist if he has noted improper fixation at the time of the gross description. If the specimen is received fresh, it should be noted if it has been allowed to dry out prior to its transportation to the laboratory.

The excised specimen should be carefully laid upon the cutting board in a manner that demonstrates the orientation of the various structures included in the dissection. The surgeon's description of the material he has submitted should be carefully matched with that received in the laboratory. Discrepancies should be noted in the description of the gross specimen and should be reported to the surgeon or the operating room supervisor.

After the specimen has been oriented on the cutting board and its components properly identified, the prosector should proceed to describe and measure its external configuration. Abnormalities in outline and consistency and unusual odors should be noted. The nature and dimensions of the attached soft tissue should also be noted.

Fragmented specimens should be placed on the cutting board and carefully examined. The specimen as aggregated on the cutting board may be measured in three dimensions, or its volume may be estimated. Either of these two estimates is relatively inaccurate. The weight of the specimen is a more accurate measure of the material received. Abnormalities or variations in consistency between various fragments should be noted and representative sections submitted. For liquid specimens, the volume, color, consistency, and the presence or absence of fixative should be noted.

Small biopsies, such as those produced by punch or aspiration techniques, are best examined under a stereoscopic microscope at which time an epithelial surface, if present, may be easily identified and the specimen properly oriented. If the technologist is not adept at handling small biopsies, it is best to place an identifying mark (India ink) on the specimen at this time to facilitate its orientation in the paraffin block. Specimens that are improperly oriented are recognized microscopically by the orientation of structures such as skin appendages or dermal papillae, which are cut in cross rather than longitudinal section. It is sometimes possible to salvage a part of the specimen by reembedding it at an angle of 90 degrees to its original orientation and then recutting the block. In many cases, however, the significant pathology will have been destroyed by the time the error is recognized. It is important to anticipate this source of error and to mark the specimen properly at the time of gross description or to instruct the technologist clearly at the time of paraffin embedding.

The most common specimen processed in a dermatopathology laboratory is cylindrical in outline and is the product of a punch biopsy. This type of specimen many range in diameter from 2 mm up to 6 or 8 mm. Punch biopsies that are 4 mm or less in diameter usually are submitted intact and are not sectioned at the cutting board. In most cases abnormalities are not apparent from the gross examination of a punch biopsy, and the pathologist's main responsibility is to record accurately the dimensions of the specimen and the presence or absence of attached subcutaneous fat.

The next most common type of specimen is one that results from an excisional or incisional biopsy. Such biopsies are usually elliptical in shape. If the biopsy is no greater than 1.5 cm wide and 2 cm long, the specimen may be bread-loaved (step-sectioned at right angles to its long axis) and submitted in toto. For biopsies of skin, it is best to turn the specimen in such a way that the epidermis is adjacent to the cutting board during sectioning. Sections may be made with a sharp scalpel, but in many cases they are best made with a sharp, single-edged razor blade. Sections through the subcutaneous fat, particularly during the examination of neoplastic processes, should be made with care. Careless sectioning may tear the subcutaneous fat away from the dermis and produce a section that is not representative of the surgical margins of excision. The margins of excision may be marked with India ink before sectioning to facilitate recognition and to document representation of margins on the microsections.

A specimen whose width is less than 7 mm in diameter, but whose length is 1 or more cm, is best bisected in its long axis. This is particularly true of specimens that are not particularly thick (less than 4 mm). Attempts to bread-loaf this type of specimen will produce sections whose widths are no greater than their thickness (vertical height). This type of section produces a problem for the technologist and is often improperly embedded.

Shave biopsies are flat and thin. An untrained technologist will often embed such a specimen on its flat surface rather than its edge. This results in microsections that are parallel to a surface. The technologist should be instructed in the proper method for orienting such a specimen.

The initial incision should be designed to best demonstrate the pathology of the excised specimen. This requires planning and thought. Perhaps because of the timidity or insecurity of many pathologists, the dissection of gross specimens at the cutting board is often incomplete. It is disturbing to review a gross specimen and to find the major pathology more or less intact with a few small radial defects where sections were removed from its edge. If the specimen has not been adequately sectioned and inspected, the examination is incomplete. A considerable amount of significant information may be obtained from the examination of the cut surface of a tumor. This information includes depth of invasion, involvement of adjacent structures, color and consistency, regional variations, invasion of blood vessels, and patterns of growth.

The appearance of the fresh cut surface of many soft tissue tumors is sufficiently characteristic to require photographic documentation of each of the representative sections. A photograph of the external surface of an intact tumor is generally meaningless and gives little information other than some idea of overall size and configuration. The cut surface and the interface between the tumor and adjacent soft tissue are important landmarks and should be accurately recorded on film. Some residents go through their entire training period without developing an appreciation for the necessity to photograph significant specimens. Part of this difficulty is that some residents never learn to recognize significant specimens from their gross characteristics. Residents who become adept in gross pathology are also likely to develop careful techniques in photography and to carefully record the appearance of significant specimens. A review of color photographs of gross specimens may occasionally reveal significant pathology that was not appreciated when the specimen was sectioned at the cutting board.

Abnormalities that are visible on the surface of the specimen should be described and the distance that separates the abnormality from the nearest margin of excision should be noted. The contours of a lesion that is visible on the external surface should be accurately described. From the character of the external configuration of a lesion it is often possible to make a distinction between basal and squamous cell neoplasms. Squamous cell tumors generally alter the epidermis and produce an abnormal amount of keratin. As a result, such a lesion often presents a central, keratin-filled crater. Basal cell tumors generally involve only the basal layer of the epidermis. As they infiltrate the dermis, they grow beneath relatively intact epidermis. As a result, the external contour of a basal cell tumor is raised, smooth and rounded. The epidermis over a basal cell carcinoma may be thinned by the underlying tumor. Tumor beneath the atrophic epidermis often produces a pearly appearance. Pigmentation is an important characteristic of the skin and its variations on the surface of the specimen should be noted and accurately described. Variations in pigmentation are characteristic features of superficial variants of melanoma (superficial spreading melanoma and lentigo maligna).

Examination under the stereoscopic scope may occasionally show the presence of abnormal lesions in the dermis at the margin of small biopsy specimens. This is particularly true of punch specimens from tumors such as basal cell carcinomas or squamous cell carcinomas. Punch specimens greater than 4 mm in diameter and elliptical specimens that are the product of incisional or excisional biopsies should be initially sectioned through a plane that best demonstrates the pathology of an externally visible lesion. Before a specimen is sectioned the information on the pathology form submitted by the clinician should be carefully reviewed. Attention should be paid to the clinical diagnosis and additional significant recorded clinical data. If the disease was clinically vesicular, the specimen should be handled with extreme care. Specimens that have been taken for the diagnosis of vesicular cutaneous diseases should not be sectioned through the vesicle. Specimens of vesicular diseases are submitted intact with instructions to the technologist to prepare multiple microsections in the hope of obtaining an intact vesicle. Since the clinician is not always careful in supplying clinical data, the external examination of punch specimens under a dissecting microscope becomes an important part of their processing. After the pathologist has assured himself from the external examination of a specimen and from a review of clinical data that sectioning will not destroy significant pathology he may proceed with the initial section. This section should be oriented perpendicular to the surface of the skin and should be directed at a level that will produce the best representation of the gross appearance of a lesion on the cut surface. It usually follows that this section will also correspond to that level where the lesion, which is visible on the external surface, extends closest to a lateral margin of excision. If the lesion is not vesicular, it is usually best to orient the specimen with the epidermis to the surface of the cutting board. The sections are then taken through the subcutaneous fat into the dermis and finally through the epidermis. The orientation of the specimen in this manner provides a firm, flat surface for sectioning. If the subcutaneous fat is placed against the cutting board, its pliability may result in sections that do not include representative portions of the deep margin. After the initial section, the gross appearance of the cut surface should be recorded. Basal cell tumors usually are lobulated and homogeneous gray. Squamous cell tumors, particularly those which keratinize, are also lobulated but show, in the center of the lobules, opaque regions that correspond to areas of keratinization. During the process of sectioning, extrusion of some of this keratin from the central portions of the cell nests may produce small cysts that are outlined by the tumor.

The pattern of the epidermis at the margin of a tumor is often an important aid in differential diagnosis. Squamous cell tumors are often associated with hyperplasia of the epidermis at the margins. Basal cell tumors are not usually characterized by alterations in the adjacent epidermis. The basal layer of the epidermis, particularly in dark-skinned patients, is pigmented and generally visible on the cut surface of a specimen. The basal layer, when pigmented, may be used as a marker in evaluating the thickness of the epidermis. Skin appendages, particularly pilosebaceous glands, may appear as opaque lobules on the cut surface of the specimen. The character or the absence of hair should be noted. Melanin appears grey or black. Blood is obvious in the fresh state, but after fixation it may appear black and be mistaken for melanin. Hemosiderin is usually brownish orange.

If a lesion is present in the demis, its margins with the adjacent dermis should be noted. It should also be noted whether the lesion in the dermis extends to the lateral or deep margins of excision.

The firmness and resilience of a specimen are sometimes an aid in diagnosis. These determinations are more applicable to the examination of fixed than fresh specimens. The value derived from determination of the resilience of the specimen is limited to specimens that possess considerable bulk. The information gained from vigorous manipulations of a small specimen will be offset by the artifacts produced by compression along a crack.

The use of Moh's paste in the treatment of skin cancer has proved to be a satisfactory method in the hands of experienced physicians. This technique finds its greatest usefulness in the management of neglected carcinomas, particularly in basal cell carcinomas that have produced extensive destruction of the soft tissues of the face. Excised specimens that have been treated with Moh's paste and submitted for frozen section are somewhat difficult to handle. The frozen sections are primarily indicated to determine the presence or absence of carcinoma. It is usually not necessary to carefully cut thin sections. Cell preservation is less than ideal following the use of Moh's paste, but it is adequate for the diagnosis of carcinoma.

SELECTION OF MATERIAL FOR MICROSECTIONING

Initial sections should be taken from the area of major or primary pathology. For tumors the initial sections should include the interface between the tumor and an epithelial surface, if one is present. Regional variations in pattern should be represented among the sections selected for microsectioning. The interface between a tumor and the adjacent normal tissue should be clearly represented. A considerable amount of information about the biology of a tumor may often be determined from its pattern of growth, particularly the manner in which it invades adjacent normal tissue. Vascular pedicles should be sectioned at the margin of excision and submitted as separate specimens. Representative sections of the involved organ away from the major pathology should also be submitted. For neoplastic processes, sections should be taken to demonstrate the routes of vascular channels.

For large tumors, sections should be taken from each significant variation in gross morphology. If the cut surface is homogeneous, a sufficient number of sections should be taken from the central portion of the tumor to give adequate histologic representation. If a variegated pattern is present on the cut surface, sections should be taken to document the variables. Significant variations in morphology also should be recorded in the gross description of the specimen.

If a tumor has been excised with a liberal margin of adjacent normal tissue, the sections taken at the interface of the tumor and the normal tissue may not include surgical margins of excision. It is usually not necessary to submit sections of the margins of excision during the examination of inflammatory processes. On the other hand, the margins of excision are important features to be examined during the study of neoplastic processes. Shaved sections from the circumference of a large specimen offer a great deal more information about the adequacy of margins of excision than radial sections. Radial sections may occasionally be indicated to demonstrate specific anatomic relationships.

Specimens that have been marked by the surgeon with sutures or dye to facilitate orientation are occasionally received. Strict attention should be paid to these markers during the gross description. Sections that include these important landmarks should be properly labeled and identified in the gross description.

Lesions containing an abundant amount of keratinized debris may exhibit an increased resistance to sectioning during preparation of the specimen. This is particularly true of epidermal cysts, and also of hyperkeratotic lesions such as calluses. Decalcification will not significantly alter the consistency of keratin unless the decalcifying solution is sufficiently acid to produce destruction of tissue. In the absence of techniques for enzymatic digestion of keratin, it is probably best to remove as much of the keratin as possible prior to submitting a specimen for processing, embedding, and microsectioning. This is particularly true of inclusion cysts. Keratinized debris within the lumen of an inclusion cyst impregnates poorly with paraffin and will often pop out of the block during attempts to microsection the specimen.

LABELING OF SECTIONS

We have already noted that sections should be representative of the lesion and should yield as much information as possible about the biology of the disease. We have also stressed that sections that demonstrate anatomic relationships or alterations of interest to the clinician may occasionally be required. Residents and sometimes practicing pathologists may occasionally go to extremes in sectioning a specimen only to have their efforts go for naught because of improper labeling. Sections that are taken to demonstrate specific features of a specimen should be clearly labeled with numbers or letters. These numbers or letters should be properly defined in the written description of the gross specimen. The description of the various labels should indicate where and of what each section is taken. The fact that sections of tissue may have clear significance for the resident or pathologist who prepared them is immaterial. They should correlate with the microscopic sections in such a way that at any time in the future a pathologist or a clinician may review the sections and make a clear interpretation of the pathology report.

In the preparation of large specimens primary emphasis should be given to the disease process and secondary emphasis should be devoted to adequacy of the margins of excision and to ancillary findings. Sections of the main portion of the lesion should be given the initial label. For a lesion such as a superficial spreading melanoma, the primary label should be assigned to those sections that are taken from the nodular portion of the lesion. Sections of lesions that are of lesser importance, such as the pigmented halo, should be assigned sequential letters or numbers. Sequential letters or numbers should then be assigned to the margins of excision, lymph nodes, and other ancillary tissues. The sequence for lettering or numbering the subsequent sections is immaterial, but should be clearly indicated in the protocol.

It is an absolute necessity to indicate clearly which of the numbered or lettered sections represent margins of excision. If radial sections are taken to include surgical margins of excision, they should be clearly labeled as such. The label should give an adequate description of the manner in which the radial section is taken so that proper orientation may be made during examination of a microscopic section.

The pathologist has an additional responsibility to indicate on the pathology report the number of sections submitted. For large specimens requiring two or more labels, the number of sections submitted under each label should be clearly indicated. This procedure assures the pathologist that material which appeared important at the time of gross sectioning has not been overlooked by the technologist during embedding. In addition, this number offers a possible check when there has been a mix-up of specimens.

The number of sections submitted in each cassette or tea bag should be recorded on a label and included in the container. This number alerts the technologist to the number of specimens included in each container. The number of containers (cassettes or tea bags) should also be recorded.

Buffered formalin (we use 4%) is a satisfactory fixative for most of the procedures required in dermatopathology. Special fixatives may be required for certain histochemical techniques but these are not a problem in routine practice of dermatopathology. Although certain substances such as mucopolysaccharides and glycogen are partially water soluble, it is usually possible to demonstrate these materials following routine fixation in formalin. Other fixatives, such as Zenker's or Bouin's, may offer advantages in the preservation of nuclear detail. These advantages are small in comparison to the problem encountered in processing tissue following the use of either of these fixatives. Bouin's fixative requires close attention to the duration of fixation.

The practice of dermatopathology often involves specimens that have been received in the mail. For this type of specimen, formalin fixation is desirable. The need for special techniques should be appreciated prior to fixation and the problems discussed between the clinician and the pathologist.

In regard to the gross description and preparation of a specimen, it should be noted that sections for microsectioning preferably should be taken after fixation. Sections that are taken from a large, fresh specimen and are subsequently fixed tend to curl and contract. This type of distortion may interfere with the proper embedding and microsectioning of the tissue. The use of techniques for rapid processing of tissue are justified primarily to facilitate and accelerate the care and management of a patient. These techniques shorten the period of hospitalization. Depending on the facilities available, it is sometimes helpful to take portions of large tumors and preserve them in a frozen state. This material may occasionally be useful if histochemical techniques are indicated after the examination of the routine sections. Consideration should also be given to the preservation of small portions in suitable fixatives for electron microscopy.

TRANSPORTATION OF SPECIMENS DURING PROCESSING.

In general, specimens are transferred from the cutting board to the tissue processor in one of two types of container. One of these is a plastic or metal cassette with openings of varying sizes, and the second is a paper tea bag. Since many specimens are small, there are obvious advantages to using the tea bag. If the metal or plastic cassettes are used it is often necessary to wrap the specimen in an absorbent paper before inserting it in the container. If this procedure is omitted, the specimen may wash through one of the openings in the cassette into the solution in the container on the tissue processor or it may wash from one cassette to a neighboring cassette and produce a disturbing mix-up in specimens. It is desirable to wrap extremely small specimens in paper even though a tea bag is used as the specimen container. Small specimens, which are impregnated with paraffin, are often difficult to recognize. It is important not to include too much tissue in a single cassette or tea bag. This error will produce poor infiltration of the tissue during processing.

PROCESSING OF SPECIMENS

Routine specimens may be processed in a routine fashion. If relatively unfixed specimens are submitted late in the day and are to be processed overnight, it is desirable to have one or more formalin baths as the initial containers on the tissue processor. The small size of many specimens requires close attention to the solutions on the tissue processor. If the tissue processor is in heavy use and solutions are not changed regularly, the tissues that will suffer most are the small ones. The result is poor tissue preservation, particularly nuclear detail. This cannot be corrected by reprocessing the tissue. Similarly, close attention should be paid to the temperature of the paraffin baths. Small specimens of skin are particularly sensitive to excessive heat.

ANTICIPATION OF SPECIAL PROCEDURES

Specimens are often received in the pathology laboratory with the request that special stains be done on the basis of clinical observations. Occasionally these observations are well founded and the requested procedures are indicated. More often they are not well founded and compliance with the clinician's request may result in needless work for the laboratory staff. It is usually wiser to request that the technologist prepare unstained sections, which are held until the routine H & E sections have been reviewed and the indicated procedures have been evaluated by the pathologist. If a request for special stains by the clinician is to be observed by the pathologist, the justification for special stains should be clearly indicated on the pathology request form. In the usual case the request is based on clinical suspicions rather than on well-founded observations, at either the clinical or the laboratory level.

The need for frozen sections is seldom a problem when dealing with material from out-patient departments. Occasionally the need arises in the management of carcinomas of the skin, particularly in relation to margins of excision. If by the use of frozen sections an attempt is made to study the margins of a large specimen for adequacy of excision, the procedure becomes extremely time-consuming. It is frustrating to the pathologist to spend a major part of his morning preparing frozen sections of margins of excision only to find that the patient has been returned to the recovery room before the task is completed. If a specimen is large and there is a problem concerning the adequacy of excision, it is usually best to request that the clinician indicate the margins that are clinically worrisome. Frozen sections at the time of surgery to outline the margins of excision are indicated procedures that are directly concerned with therapeutic decisions. If the margin of excision is so close that the interpretation of the slide as positive or negative depends upon which of two opposite surfaces is sectioned, the surgical margin is inadequate.

A frozen section is indicated if a therapeutic decisions is involved. Frozen sections are abused by both the clinician and the pathologist. The clinician abuses the rationale of a frozen section if he orders it routinely, even when therapeutic decisions are not involved. Occasionally the frozen section assumes the proportions of a prestige item. In the eyes of the clinician the value of the frozen section may be severely limited if the pathologist commonly either offers arbitrary diagnoses or is unwilling to render a diagnosis.

The use of metachromatic dyes on frozen sections followed by the application of a cover slip over a drop of glycerin or water is a satisfactory technique for rapid staining of frozen sections. In general, considerably more nuclear detail is preserved with metachromatic dyes than with formalin fixation and rapid staining with hematoxylin and eosin. For problem cases it may be advisable to use both techniques, preserving the H & E stained sections for the hospital files.

It is the responsibility of the pathologist to obtain some assurance from the surgeon that additional material for permanent sections will be forthcoming before doing a frozen section on a small specimen. On permanent sections, the artifacts induced in tissue by freezing and thawing may severely hamper the ability of the pathologist to render a specific diagnosis.

Competence in the diagnosis of gross specimens facilitates the selection of areas to be submitted for frozen section. One of the pitfalls in performing a frozen section is the selection of tissue that is not representative of the main tumor. This is sometimes an unavoidable source of error, but may be minimized by awareness of the possibility and by developing competence in the recognition of gross characteristics. Such competence also generally facilitates the interpretation of a frozen section.

Prior to radical surgery, it is usually preferable to have an accurate diagnosis on tissue that has been routinely processed. Although it is frequently possible to make an accurate diagnosis from a frozen section of a small portion of a tumor, there are pitfalls if complete reliance is placed on this technique. A frozen section of a needle biopsy of a mesenchymal tumor is probably not indicated.

SPECIAL STAINS

The following stains are of value as relatively routine procedures in dermatopathology and in general may be used on formalin-fixed tissue.

1. Periodic acid Schiff.
    a. Without diastase. For glycogen and mucopolysaccharides.
    b. With diastase digestion and with hematoxylin counterstain. This is a satisfactory stain for fungi and has the advantage of removing much of the nonspecific PAS positive material that often is present in inflammatory processes.
2. Gridley stain-fungi.

3. Gomori silver methenamine stain-fungi. Difficult to control and may obscure morphology of the fungus. A Gridley stain is generally preferred but Gomori's stain is useful in old granulomas containing dead organisms.
4. Giemsa. This stain demonstrates metachromatic substances, particularly mast cell granules. It also is a good stain for demonstrating eosinophiles. (Acid orcein and giemsa stain is a useful variation.)
5. Alcian blue stain. For demonstration of acid mucopolysaccharides, particularly in dermal mucinoses and in alopecia mucinosa.
6. Reticulum stain (Wilder's or Snook's method).
7. Prussian blue reaction for iron.
8. Fontana Masson stain for demonstration of melanin.
9. Acid-fast stains (Ziehl-Neelsen's and Fite's stain).
10. Gram stain.
11. Congo Red for demonstration of amyloid. This stain is apparently difficult to control and often hard to interpret. Positive staining may be enhanced by examination under polarized light. The positive areas exhibit a green dichroism under polarized light.
12. Crystal violet. This metachromatic stain may be used to demonstrate acid mucopolysaccharides and amyloid. It is a satisfactory stain for mast cells and for demonstration of tissue mucins in the various mucinoses. The metachromasia of amyloid may be enhanced by examination under polarized light.
13. Warthin-Starry. This stain may be used to demonstrate spirochetes but is especially useful to demonstrate Donovan bodies in granuloma inguinale. Donovan bodies may also be demonstrated with Giemsa stain.
14. PTAH (phosphotungstic acid hematoxylin). For fibrin, inclusion bodies, elastica of reticular dermis (does not stain that in papillary dermis), and myelin.
15. Verhoeff-van Gieson. For connective tissues, especially elastica.
16. Orcein. For elastica.
17. Masson's trichrome. For connective tissues (superior to one-step trichrome), smooth muscle, etc.
18. Bodian stain. For neurites, myofibrils.
19. Colloidal iron. For connective tissue.

There are definite advantages in having multiple tissue sections of a biopsy specimen represented on a slide. Two or more ribbons containing multiple sections can be placed on a slide. To facilitate this procedure, the margins of the paraffin block should be tapered from the back to the face. By limiting the surface area of the face of the block it is possible to crowd several sections into a ribbon. Since most pathologists manually move a slide over the stage of a microscope rather than relying upon a mechanical stage, and in the process move the slide from left to right (or vice versa), it is an advantage to have a relatively straight ribbon oriented along the longitudinal axis of the glass slide. There are advantages if the longitudinal axis of the epidermis parallels the longitudinal axis of the ribbon. This requirement should be considered when the paraffin block is oriented on the microtome.

Chapter 5

Histopathology

MICROSCOPIC ANATOMY AND REACTION PATTERNS OF THE SKIN

The interpretation of a histologic section of the skin involves a systematic study of the epidermis, the skin appendages, the dermis, and the panniculus adiposus. The dermis is composed of the adventitial dermis and the reticular dermis. The former is composed of the papillary dermis, the perifollicular connective tissue sheaths, and the adventitia of blood vessels. Two of these components (papillary and perifollicular dermis) support and interact with epithelium. The relationships between these two connective tissue components and their epithelia are so intimate that it is difficult to discuss one without a consideration of the other.

At the histologic level, a study of the epidermis requires that attention be paid to the keratin layer (stratum corneum), the granular layer (stratum granulosum), the intermediate or stratified layer (stratum malpighii), and the basal layer (stratum basalis). Although the basal layer is also considered to be a germinal layer from which the regenerating cells replenish the overlying layers, its major function is probably the maintainance and preservation of the interface between epithelium and dermis. The distribution and character of melanocytes in the epidermis should also be noted.

The fibers of the papillary dermis, a narrow zone of connective tissue between the epidermis and the reticular dermis, are delicate and randomly arranged. They are associated with delicate elastic fibers that branch and extend into the dermal papillae, which are projections at the surface of the papillary dermis that interdigitate with epidermal processes (rete ridges). The elastic fibers of the papillary dermis are PTAH (phosphotungstic acid hematoxylin) negative. The perifollicular sheaths, which are extensions of the papillary dermis, are responsive to the growth cycles of hair follicles. At the extremity of a growing hair follicle, the bulb induces a special alteration in the adjacent sheath which is called the papilla. The latter is a localized cellular area of well-vascularized, mucinous connective tissue. Sebaceous glands are glandular outpouchings from the wall of follicles. They are usually located in the middermis and may be used as markers to determine levels of invasion in the evaluation of skin tumors.

The reticular dermis is a mat of coarse, interwoven bundles of collagen fibers. Neurovascular bundles course through the reticular dermis. A lymphatic plexus is also present, but normally is inconspicuous. The elastic fibers of the reticular dermis are coarse, segmented, and branched. They follow the direction of the adjacent collagen bundles and are PTAH positive. Septa that are extensions of the reticular dermis surround lobules of adipose tissue in the panniculus adiposus.

Sweat glands are coiled, secretory glands that are situated at the lower margin of the dermis. They are surrounded by adipose tissue. The glands have a double layer of epithelium. They communicate through excretory ducts with the surface of the skin. The ducts are lined by squamous epithelium. Their lumina are outlined by birefringent, hyaline cuticles. Apocrine glands are limited in distribution and are most numerous in the axillae and in the genital areas. Their secretory cells have an abundant amount of granular cytoplasm. Characteristically, they show decapitation secretion. Their excretory ducts are similar to those of eccrine glands, but may empty into the upper portions of hair follicles rather than the surface of the epidermis.

The panniculus adiposus is a specialized fascial layer composed of lobules of closely aggregated lipocytes. The lobules are supported by fibrous septa that extend from the lower margin of the dermis to the superficial layer of the deep fascia. They are supplied by a nutrient artery with venous drainage to the periphery of the lobules. Interference with the arterial supply produces diffuse alterations in the involved lobules. Interference with venous drainage produces changes in the fibrous septa and in the lobules at their interface with the septa. In the evaluation of disease of the panniculus adiposus attention should be paid to its blood vessels, its lobules of lipocytes, and its fibrous septa.

There are distinctive features of keratinizing squamous epithelium that are evident in both inflammatory and neoplastic diseases. During periods of rapid turnover of cells, the process is characterized by an increased proportion of poorly keratinized cells that have the cytoplasmic characteristics of adjacent basal cells and by a defective formation of the granular layer. The end result is a product that is distinctly different from that normally produced. The keratin layer that results from this faulty pathway is composed of plump, acidophilic, keratinized cells that contain pyknotic nuclei (parakeratosis).

In some lesions, faulty keratinization is indicated by hyperplasia of the granular layer and thickening of the keratin layer. Usually this keratin layer is composed of compactly arranged, flattened, anuclear keratinocytes (hyperkeratosis).

In many inflammatory and neoplastic processes involving keratinocytes, faulty keratinization of individual cells (dyskeratosis) is a prominent feature. Dyskeratosis is indicated not only by premature keratinization
(appearing in intermediate layer), but also by faulty aggregation of keratin
(readily demonstrated by intense birefringence when examined under
polarized light).

In dyskeratotic processes, there is often faulty cohesion of the diseased
keratinocytes (acantholysis). Acantholysis may be a prominent feature
of some examples of basal keratinocytic dysplasia. It is also a feature of
some squamous cell carcinomas and may be associated with the production of a mucinous matrix that accumulates in the clefts that result from
the defects in cellular cohesion.

The patterns of inflammatory reactions in the dermis are limited. Most
inflammatory processes are limited to the superficial vascular plexus. The
papillary dermis is usually involved. Varying patterns of epidermal reactions may accompany inflammation in the dermis.

A less common but more distinctive pattern of dermal inflammation
is characterized by perivenular infiltrates that extend from the upper to
the lower portion of the reticular dermis. The papillary dermis is relatively
spared. This pattern of inflammation may be seen in the clinical settings
of lupus erythematosus, polymorphic light eruption, and persistent ery-
themas (erythema annulare centrifugum, etc.). It is commonly associated
with damage to collagen in the reticular dermis. Occasionally it is difficult
to decide if the process is primarily a collagenosis rather than a lymphocytic
vasculitis.

The histologic patterns of dermal vasculitides are basically the same
as those seen in other organs. Clinically they are sometimes fixed, chronic
processes that paradoxically show histologic features of an acute process.
Erythema elevatum diutinum and granuloma faciale are examples of
"fixed," necrotizing vasculitides. Thrombotic and necrotizing vasculitides
that are relatively free of inflammatory cells may occur in some cutaneous
syndromes. This reaction is seen in so-called livedo vasculitis (livedo
reticularis, atrophie blanche, seasonal ulcers) and may be symptomatic of
collagen diseases. The vascular changes are reminiscent of those seen
in the kidneys, the periadrenal fat, and the pancreas in malignant
nephrosclerosis.

It is not possible to discuss the reaction patterns of the dermal connective tissue or the panniculus adiposus in this book. The changes in
the skin in various systemic disorders may be compared to those in other
organ systems. Often they are a problem only because archaic terminology
may offer little insight into the basic nature of the process.

POINTS OF EMPHASIS IN HISTOLOGIC DESCRIPTIONS

In the interpretation of histologic sections of cutaneous tumors, there are points of emphasis other than cell type, differentiation, size of tumor, and pattern of growth (pushing or infiltrating margins). The interpretation of an incisional biopsy specimen is concerned primarily with classification of the tumor. If the tumor is of epithelial origin, it should be noted whether the site of origin is apparent on the sections examined. This observation also is pertinent to the interpretation of excisional biopsy specimens and may alert the clinician to the possibility of a cutaneous metastasis or a recurrent lesion rather than primary tumor. The depth of dermal invasion is also pertinent. The sebaceous glands may be used as a marker for the middermis. The sweat glands are markers for the lower limit of the dermis. If the specimen is from a sun-exposed surface, then actinically altered connective tissue may be present in the dermis. This material accumulates primarily in the upper portion of the reticular dermis and tends to spare the papillary dermis. If an epithelial process has compressed, but has not extended into or through this band of altered connective tissue, then significant invasion probably has not occurred. Blood vessel, lymphatic, or nerve sheath invasion should be searched for and noted in the report.

THE EVALUATION OF EPIDERMOID CARCINOMA OF THE SKIN

The following variants of cutaneous epidermoid carcinoma may be recognized:

1. actinic
2. bowenoid or arsenical
3. scar
4. de novo

The first three variants are usually preceded by keratinocytic dysplasia.

Basal Keratinocytic Dysplasia

The most common type of epidermal keratinocytic dysplasia is induced by actinic irradiation. The dysplastic process affects primarily the basal layer of the epidermis, and in some examples is confined to this zone. Atypical changes may involve the entire thickness of the epidermis, but the process usually is less severe in the intermediate and the granular layer than it is in the basal layer (Fig. 5-1). Often the zone of dysplasia

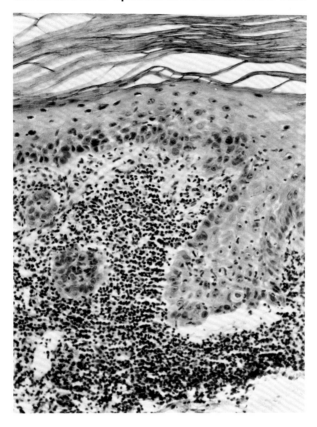

Fig. 5-1. Moderate basal keratinocytic dysplasia showing atypical changes more or less confined to the basal portion of the epidermis. A bandlike infiltrate of chronic inflammatory cells is present in the dermis, and in one area hugs an elongated rete ridge. In this area a cleft has formed between the epithelium and the dermal infiltrate.

involving the basal layer is separated from the overlying intermediate layer by a cleft (acantholysis). This peculiar pattern of growth implies that the basal layer of the epidermis may be functionally distinct from the intermediate layer. In those examples in which the basal layer is dysplastic and the overlying intermediate layer is cytologically normal, the former does not appear to make a contribution to the latter, nor does the latter seem to require the presence of a basal layer to replenish itself. This form of keratinocytic dysplasia is spoken of as actinic or solar keratosis. It is premalignant but its invasive counterpart is generally a tumor with little biologic potenial. It is almost invariably associated with actinic damage to dermal connective tissue.

Histopathology

Intermediate Keratinocytic Dysplasia

The second form of keratinocytic dysplasia is not closely associated with actinic damage. It is characterized by dysplastic changes that are most evident in the intermediate layer. In contrast to basal keratinocytic dysplasia, the intermediate variant is usually hyperplastic and has a significantly increased mitotic rate (Fig. 5-2). Abnormal mitoses are usually present. Loss of polarity and premature keratinization of individual cells are important features. The rete ridges are usually elongated. In contrast, the rete ridges in a lesion showing basal keratinocytic dysplasia are usually effaced. The intermediate keratinocytic dysplasias seldom show significant alterations in the basal layer. Clinically they correspond to lesions that are classified as Bowen's disease. Similar lesions occasionally may arise on a background of actinic damage (Fig. 5-3).

The differentiation between basal keratinocytic dysplasia and intermediate keratinocytic dysplasia is important. Tumors that arise from

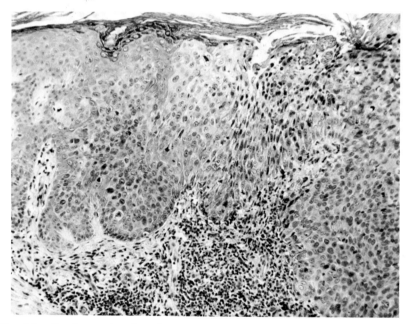

Fig. 5-2. Carcinoma in situ showing the pattern of intermediate keratinocytic dysplasia. A relatively intact row of basal cells surrounds the atypical keratinocytes in most areas. The atypism extends from above the basal portion of the epidermis to the horny layer. A bandlike infiltrate of inflammatory cells is present in the dermis. In the area in which the infiltrate hugs the epithelium, the basal layer has been partially destroyed.

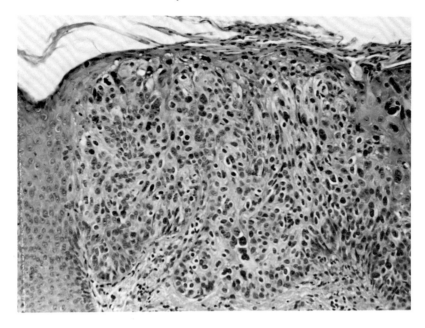

Fig. 5-3. Actinically induced intermediate keratinocytic dysplasia (carcinoma in situ) showing changes similar to those seen in the de novo lesion in Fig. 5-2. The atypical changes are more or less confined to the intermediate zone of the epidermis. The basal layer is relatively intact and shows little or no atypism.

lesions of the intermediate type of dysplasia tend to be aggressive and to have a relatively high incidence of metastasis. There is also evidence that they are associated with an increased incidence of internal malignancies. Tumors that arise from lesions showing dysplasia of the basal type are relatively indolent and seldom metastasize.

Primary Carcinoma of the Skin

The histologic evaluation of a primary carcinoma of the skin is based on one or more of the following features:

1. depth of invasion
2. differentiation
3. stromal response
4. inflammatory response
5. antecedent lesion, if any
6. site of origin

7. blood vessel invasion
8. nerve sheath invasion
9. configuration of tumor
   a. pushing margin
   b. infiltrating margin

There are three significant levels of dermal invasion. The first level is the papillary dermis. If the infiltrating cords of tumor cells have extended no deeper than the papillary dermis, the prognosis and the clinical management are essentially those of an actinic keratosis (basal keratinocytic dysplasia). If the cells have infiltrated into but not beyond the reticular dermis, the likelihood of metastasis is remote, especially for those tumors that have their origin on a background of actinic damage. In the reticular dermis, the tumor has access to peripheral nerves. In this location occult extensions beyond the margins of excision may serve as foci for regrowth of tumor. The boundary for the third level is the lower margin of the reticular dermis (panniculus adiposus or skeletal muscle). The incidence of metastasis at this level is higher than that of the second level.

The differentiation of keratinocytic tumors is prognostically significant, but probably is not a prime determinant. The evaluation of differentiation is based on nuclear atypism and on the relative proportion of keratinizing and nonkeratinizing cells. If atypism is confined to a single peripheral layer and if the bulk of each cell nest is composed of keratinizing cells that show minimal nuclear atypism, the tumor is well differentiated (Grade I). If a peripheral layer of nonkeratinizing, markedly atypical cells forms the bulk of each cell nest but central areas of keratinization are present, the tumor is moderately differentiated (Grade II). If the cell nests are composed of poorly differentiated cells with only scattered single cells showing evidence of keratinization, it is poorly differentiated (Grade III).

THE STROMAL RESPONSES TO EPITHELIAL TUMORS OF THE SKIN

General Stromal Responses

The stromal responses to epithelial tumors of the skin are variable but are related to the nature of the tumor cells. They may be divided into the following categories:

1. reactive stroma
2. induced stroma

3. granulation tissue stroma
4. sclerosing stroma
5. amyloid stroma
6. refractory stroma

The basic response of connective tissue to an infiltrating carcinoma is the reactive stroma. It is not peculiar to the skin but is seen in various tissues and organs. It is characterized by elongated fibroblastic spindle cells that parallel the outlines of the tumor cell nests (Fig. 5-4). The reactive stromal cells are separated from their neighbors by rigid, relatively straight bundles of collagen. The reactive stroma is the characteristic response of the dermis to an actively growing, infiltrating epidermoid carcinoma. Occasionally the stroma is myxomatous (Fig. 5-5).

The induced stroma is a special form of connective tissue that is myxomatous or fibrous. Its fibers are delicate and randomly arranged (Fig. 5-6). In its myxomatous phase, the induced stroma may be compared to the induced stroma of the hair papilla (Fig. 5-7). In its fibrous phase,

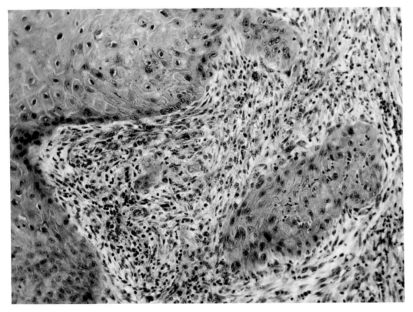

Fig. 5-4. Keratoacanthoma showing reactive stroma surrounding nests of infiltrating keratinocytes. The infiltrating tumor shows slight keratinocytic dysplasia at its advancing margin. The basal layer is no longer recognizable in many of the areas in which the tumor cells are in contact with the reactive stroma.

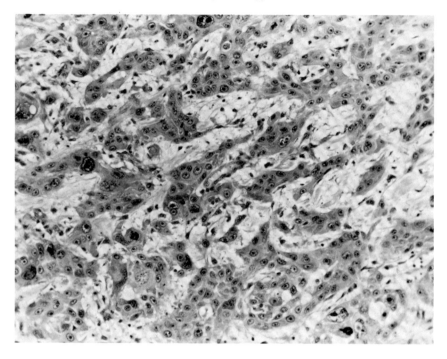

Fig. 5-5. Infiltrating poorly differentiated epidermoid carcinoma showing a reactive stroma that has myxomatous qualities. The tumor cells are not keratinizing. This uniform absence of keratinized debris qualifies the lesion as poorly differentiated squamous cell carcinoma.

it may be compared to the papillary or perifollicular dermis. The induced stroma is an integral part of the tumor and extends in continuity with the tumor cells from the adventitial dermis (Fig. 5-6). The induced stroma is a characteristic response of the dermis to usual type of basal cell "carcinoma." Its presence in a basal cell "carcinoma" is evidence of differentiation. Basal cell tumors with uniformly induced stroma tend to remain confined to the dermis. They are organoid tumors that are unlikely to metastasize. As an explanation for the relative absence of metastasis from basal cell carcinomas, it has been proposed that the tumor cells do not have the ability to induce a suitable stroma in the foreign environment of a metastatic site. In the absence of a suitable induced stroma, the tumor cells do not survive. Not all basal cell tumors induce a stroma. Some stimulate a reactive stroma (Fig. 5-8). These forms of basal cell tumors do not respect the boundaries of the dermis, may extensively infiltrate soft tissue, and may metastasize (Fig. 5-9). Basal cell tumors with a reactive stroma are properly classified as basal cell carcinomas. Many of the so-called

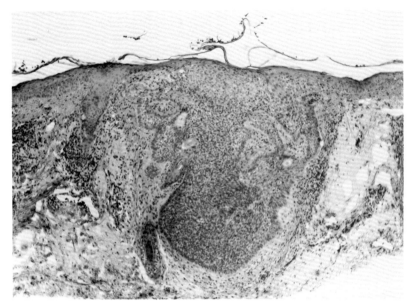

Fig. 5-6. Small basal cell carcinoma with induced stroma. The induced stroma surrounds the nests of proliferating cells and is continuous with the papillary dermis.

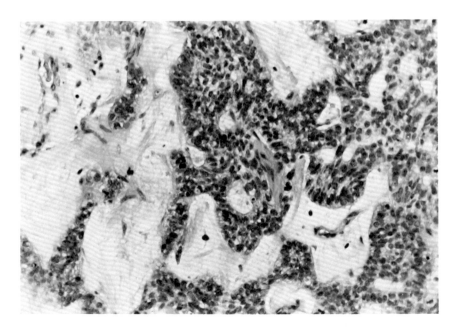

Fig. 5-7. Basal cell carcinoma with myxomatous induced stroma. The stroma is hypocellular and contains scattered small vessels.

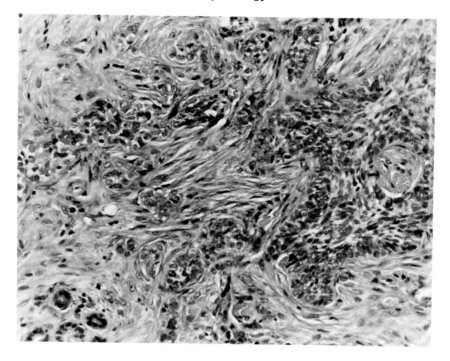

Fig. 5-8. Basal cell carcinoma with reactive stroma. The tumor has extended to the level of the sweat glands.

metatypical carcinomas are examples of basal cell carcinomas with reactive stroma.

Rare examples of basal cell "carcinoma" that have an induced stroma are additionally characterized by the formation of coarse hyalinized bundles of collagen (Fig. 5-10). These broad bands of collagen are reminiscent of those seen in keloids.

Adenoid cystic carcinomas of sweat gland origin have an induced stroma. The mixed tumor of sweat gland origin is characterized by an induced and metaplastic stroma.

A variety of organoid epithelial tumors of the skin are confined to or are associated with a localized hyperplasia of the papillary dermis. Seborrheic keratoses, inverted follicular keratoses, tricholemmomas, and skin tags are included in this group. These lesions may be included in the category of cutaneous epithelial tumors with induced stroma.

The granulation tissue stroma is seen in some epidermoid carcinomas, particularly papillary variants. It may also be seen in carcinomas arising on the hands and feet and is common as a regional variation in keratoa-

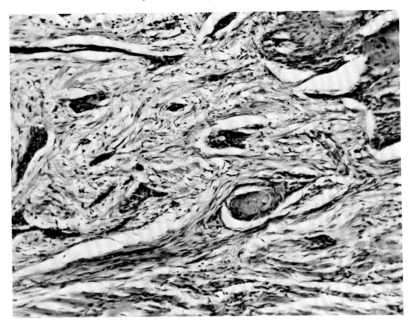

Fig. 5-9. Baso-squamous carcinoma infiltrating skeletal muscle at deep margin of dermis. The tumor is composed in part of basal cells having peripheral palisading of the nuclei. In addition, there are clefts between the nests of tumor cells and the stroma. These features are in keeping with those seen in basal cell carcinoma, but the tumor is additionally distinguished by areas of squamous cell differentiation and by an aggressive pattern of growth. The tumor has infiltrated a nerve near the lower margin of the field and has stimulated a reactive stroma. It metastasized to regional lymph nodes.

canthomas. Some benign skin appendage tumors have granulation tissue stromas. Included in the latter group are eccrine poroma and the pale cell acanthoma of Degos. This type of stroma is characterized by clusters of tortuous thick-walled capillaries in a delicate, relatively clear matrix (Fig. 5-11). Granulation tissue stromas are common at the advancing margins of those melanomas that grow in an expansile fashion.

Stromas of a somewhat different character are seen in basaloid tumors showing sweat gland differentiation (i.e., eccrine spiradenoma and eccrine cylindroma). In these tumors the specialized stroma is hyalinized.

Sclerosing stromas are densely fibrous and poorly cellular. They are characteristically seen in sweat gland tumors that are composed of squamous and clear cells (eccrine acrospiroma or clear cell myoepithelioma). Rarely lesions in the latter group show one or more areas in which small nests of cells are associated with a reactive stroma (Fig. 5-12). This pat-

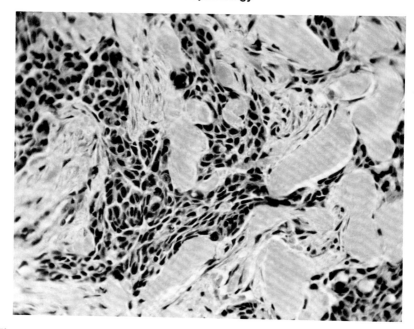

Fig. 5-10.   Basal cell carcinoma with "keloidal" reaction in stroma.

tern is not proof of carcinomatous change and its significance is not known. Almost certainly its presence is evidence of active growth. Some histologically benign eccrine acrospiromas have metastasized. Perhaps the presence of a reactive stroma is correlated with an increased likelihood of metastasis, but this is not proved.

Syringomatous basal cell carcinoma is characterized by elongated tortuous cords of basal cells. Some of the cords of cells that have a doubled layered wall surrounding a lumen bear a strong resemblance to sweat ducts. This tumor does not induce a readily recognized stroma. Its stroma is scanty, and in the dermis the tumor cells appear to have adapted to interstitial spaces between collagen bundles of the reticular dermis (Fig. 5-13*a,b*). The reticular dermis is thickened. This variant of basal cell carcinoma is aggressive. It extends beyond the confines of the dermis into the panniculus adiposus and into deep soft tissue and bone. In the panniculus adiposus its thin sheath of induced stroma is usually apparent.

Amyloid deposits may occasionally be a feature of the stroma of cutaneous epithelial tumors. These deposits are more commonly found in the stroma of basal cell carcinomas, particularly those with an induced

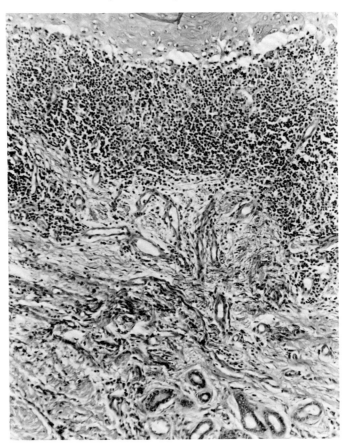

Fig. 5-11. Deep margin of keratoacanthoma showing granulation tissue stroma between tumor cells and underlying reticular dermis. The granulation tissue is heavily infiltrated with inflammatory cells, which hug the nests of tumor cells to produce a lichenoid pattern with focal destruction of keratinocytes.

stroma (Fig. 5-14), but may also be seen in benign epithelial tumors such as seborrheic keratoses and in carcinoma in situ of the intermediate type (Fig. 5-15). The amyloid deposits are almost invariably globular and occasionally extend to the interface between the tumor cells and their stroma. Often the amyloid deposits are associated with pigmented dendritic cells. These deposits are similar to those seen in the conditions known as lichen and macular amyloidosis. There is some evidence that the deposits in the latter process may be of epithelial origin. Although the his-

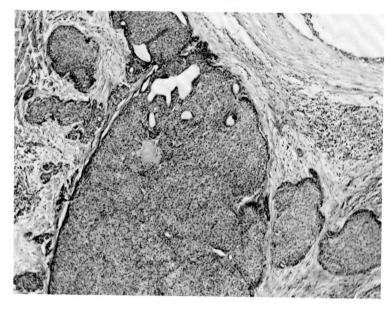

Fig. 5-12. Eccrine acrospiroma showing solid and cystic patterns. Areas of glandular differentiation are present in the solid portion. Small nests of basaloid cells extend into a reactive stroma.

togenesis of these deposits is uncertain, they are regularly associated with epithelial lesions. The term epithelial amyloidosis is descriptive of this variant. These deposits of amyloid are not associated with systemic disease. They appear to be associated with atrophy of tumor cells in regions of contact with the amyloid. In carcinoma in situ these deposits may be prominent in areas of regression and may be evidence of immune processes.

The refractory stroma is a descriptive term for a defective stromal response to an infiltrating epithelial tumor. The characteristic features of this reaction pattern are:

1. rapid growth,
2. extension of an epithelial neoplasm into the dermis without prior dissolution or replacement of preexisting connective tissue components by a reactive stroma,
3. fragmentation of dermal components by the infiltrating tumor,
4. extrusion of fragmented connective tissue fibers through the interstices of the invading tumor cells to the surface of the skin,
5. complete or partial destruction of tumor cells at cessation of refractory period.

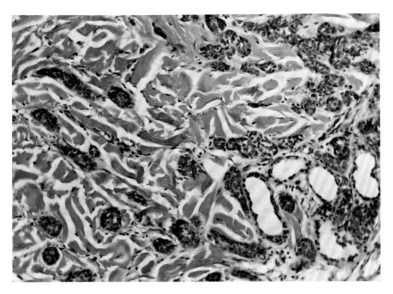

Fig. 5-13*a*. Syringomatous basal cell carcinoma showing cords and tubules, some of which are lined by a double layer of cells. There is minimal stromal response.

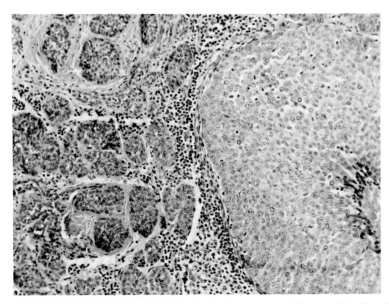

Fig. 5-13*b*. Metastasis to regional lymph node from tumor illustrated in Fig. 5-13*a*. The tumor is basaloid and has a pattern resembling that seen in some eccrine acrospiromas.

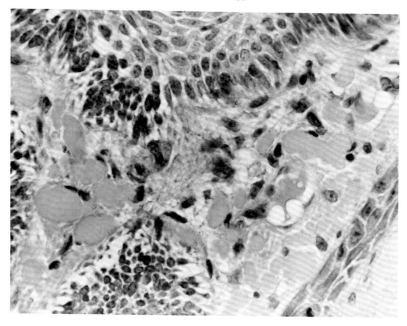

Fig. 5-14. Basal cell carcinoma with induced stroma containing deposits of amyloid. The material is positive with congo red stain and with crystal violet stain. This form of amyloidosis is not uncommon in association with basal cell carcinomas that have an induced stroma. Characteristically, the material accumulates in globules and is commonly associated with numerous dendritic cells.

Keratinocytic Tumors with Refractory Stroma (Keratoacanthoma)

It is obvious from the features enumerated above that the epidermal tumors with refractory stromas are representative of the group of tumors classified as keratoacanthomas. The usual epidermoid carcinoma of the skin evolves slowly. During its growth it stimulates a reactive stroma that replaces the dermis in advance of the infiltrating cords of epithelial cells. A keratoacanthoma evolves rapidly and floods the dermis (Figs. 5-16 and 5-17) before the dermis can react to produce a reactive or granulation tissue stroma (probably sometime after the initial 6- to 8-week period of rapid growth). The usual histologic features of keratoacanthoma are summarized in Table 5-1.

In any large group of keratoacanthomas there is a wide histologic spectrum that ranges from lesions that are cytologically benign (Fig. 5-18) to those that are indistinguishable from epidermoid carcinomas (Fig. 5-19). There may be significant variations in pattern in a single lesion (Fig. 5-19;

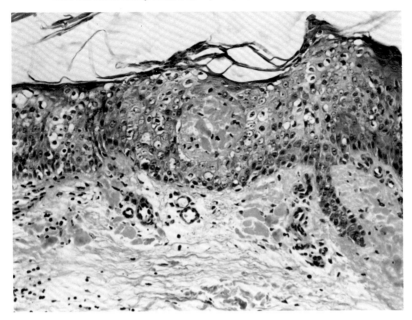

Fig. 5-15. Intermediate keratinocytic dysplasia (carcinoma in situ) showing globular deposits of amyloid in a thickened papillary dermis. A localized collection of similar material is present in the epidermis in the central portion of the field. This may represent amyloid within the dermis in a rete ridge that has been cut in cross section but the material appears to lie within the epidermis.

see also Figs. 6-79 and 6-80). In the latter group, it is not possible to predict with any degree of certainty whether the tumor will spontaneously resolve or will persist and enter a chronic growth phase which is indistinguishable from that of the ordinary epidermoid carcinoma. In most instances the keratoacanthoma appears to be an acute, benign, self-limited disease. Some of the lesions, however, will persist and enter a chronic phase characterized by slowly progressive growth and aggressive behavior. These two phases might be spoken of as acute and chronic carcinoma (Fig. 5-20). The ordinary carcinoma of the skin is also a chronic lesion but is not preceded by an acute phase. These growth patterns are indicated in the graph (Fig. 5-21). Although nerve sheath invasion has been described in keratoacanthomas, it is an unusual feature (Fig. 5-22). Blood vessel invasion occasionally has been noted. (Fig. 5-23). Caution should be exercised in the diagnosis of keratoacanthoma for lesions that have extended to the third level of invasion (through the reticular dermis) and for lesions arising on mucocutaneous junctions (Fig. 5-24). Once the histologic features of keratoacanthoma have been recognized the

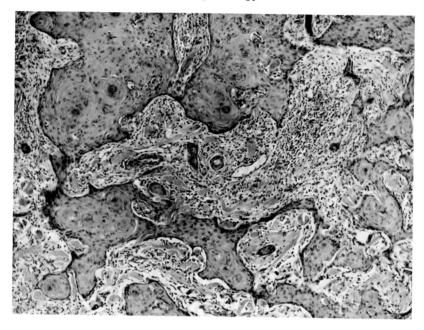

Fig. 5-16. Lateral margin of actively growing keratoacanthoma showing extension of nests of tumor cells into reticular dermis. Collagen bundles are preserved and have been extruded into the interstices of the invading epithelium. An infiltrate of inflammatory cells is present but the tumor has not stimulated a significant reactive stroma. There is minimal keratinocytic dysplasia in the advancing margin of this tumor.

lesion should be additionally qualified as to degree of keratinocytic dysplasia (slight, moderate, or marked). Cytologically, keratoacanthomas with marked keratinocytic dysplasia are indistinguishable from epidermoid carcinomas. Some melanomas and occasional epidermoid carcinomas that actively infiltrate the dermis at their advancing margin also are characterized by stromal refractoriness (Fig. 5-25).

THE REACTIONS AT THE INTERFACE BETWEEN CUTANEOUS CARCINOMAS AND THEIR STROMA

The interface between epithelium of the skin and the adjacent dermis is characterized by a condensation of matrix that is spoken of as the basement membrane or as basal lamina. At the level of the light microscope this zone is characterized by a membranous condensation of reticulin fibers and by a PAS positive matrix. In the evaluation of dermal invasion by cutaneous

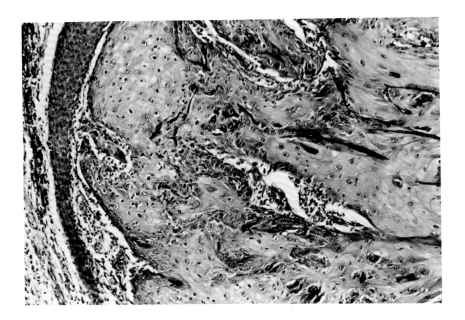

Fig. 5-17. Invading lateral margin of actively growing keratoacanthoma showing extrusion of altered connective tissue into the interstices of the invading keratinocytes. Clusters of acute inflammatory cells are present in the nests of tumor cells and may represent a response to extruded connective tissue. VVG.

Table 5-1
Clinical and Histologic Features of Keratoacanthoma

1. Rapid growth over a period of weeks.
2. Spontaneous involution over a period of months.
3. Cup-shaped lesion with a central, keratin-filled crater.
4. "Flooding" of the dermis with hyperplastic squamous cells.
5. Prominent inflammatory reaction in the surrounding dermis.
6. Intraepithelial "abscesses."
7. Lesion composed of large squamous cells with abundant, watery, pale cytoplasm.
8. Scarring of the dermis following involution.
9. "Buttress" that is formed of epidermal folds at margins of central crater.
10. Participation of pilosebaceous and sweat duct epithelium in the localized area of epithelial hyperplasia (field phenomena).
11. Dissolution of squamous cell nests and isolation of individual cells by an inflammatory infiltrate.
12. Variable atypism in the advancing margins of the infiltrating cell nests (one-third of these tumors cytologically indistinguishable from carcinoma).
13. Invasion usually limited in depth to the level of the sweat glands.

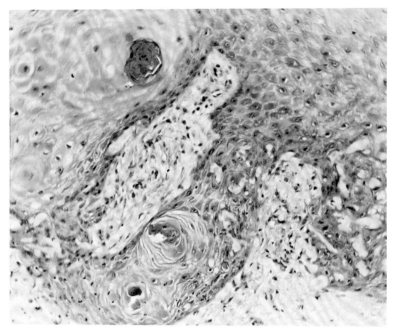

Fig. 5-18. Lateral margin of actively growing keratoacanthoma showing extrusion of altered connective tissue into the interstices of the invading tumor cells. There is evidence of a reactive stroma with the proliferation of blood vessels and fibrocytes.

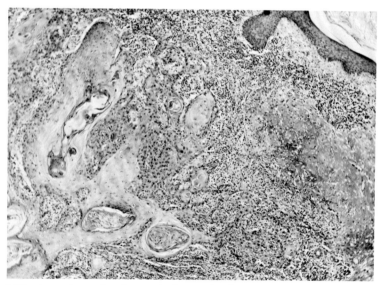

Fig. 5-19. Lateral margin of an actively growing keratoacanthoma showing a degree of keratinocytic dysplasia indistinguishable from that seen in cutaneous epidermoid carcinomas. An inflamed reactive stroma separates the tumor from actinically damaged connective tissue of the dermis.

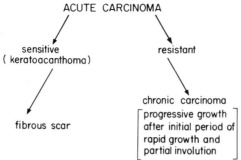

ACUTE CARCINOMA

sensitive
(keratoacanthoma)

resistant

fibrous scar

chronic carcinoma
⌈progressive growth⌉
│after initial period of│
│rapid growth and│
⌊partial involution⌋

Fig. 5-20. The term acute carcinoma characterizes those forms of rapidly growing cutaneous tumors that are derived from squamous epithelium and show the clinical characteristics of keratoacanthomas. Within this group of lesions there are tumors that are cytologically benign, tumors that are borderline in atypism, and tumors that are cytologically malignant. Most of the lesions in the category of acute carcinoma will prove to be sensitive to the host's defenses and will spontaneously involute, forming a fibrous scar. The term keratoacanthoma was developed to describe this type of lesion. A small number of acute carcinomas prove to be resistant to the host's defenses and, after partial involution, show continued growth and may eventually metastasize. The sensitive tumors result in the formation of a fibrous scar. The resistant tumors evolve into chronic lesions that are otherwise indistinguishable from squamous cell carcinomas of the skin.

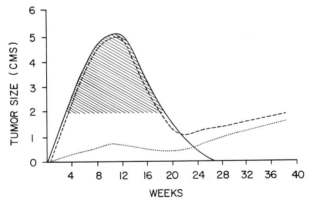

Fig. 5-21. Chronic resistant carcinomas are represented by the dotted line. Acute sensitive carcinomas are represented by a solid line. Acute resistant carcinomas are represented by a broken line. Chronic resistant carcinomas are characterized by relatively slow increase in size over several months. Acute carcinomas are characterized by an explosive onset with rapid growth over several weeks. This is followed by a period of involution. In the acute sensitive form, the involution is generally completed within 6 months. Acute resistant carcinomas may also show involution, but it is generally incomplete and is followed by a phase that more or less corresponds to that of chronic progressive carcinomas. The shaded area represents the period in which acute sensitive and acute resistant carcinomas overlap in their clinical behavior. During this period it is not possible to predict which of the acute carcinomas will prove to be resistant and which will persist as chronic carcinomas. This problem can be answered only by the biologic evolution of the tumor over a period of time and cannot be predicted for every case from the histologic examination.

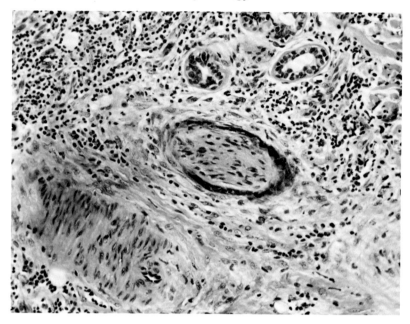

Fig. 5-22. Deep margin of keratoacanthoma showing nerve sheath invasion. The tumor was clinically aggressive and recurred twice. It arose on a mucocutaneous junction (lip) and had extended into skeletal muscle. The lesion showed a minimal amount of keratinocytic dysplasia.

tumors, emphasis has been placed on the presence or absence of a basement membrane about the nests of tumor cells. The absence of a basement membrane is generally accepted as evidence of invasive growth. The significance of a defective basement membrane in areas of invasion is not known. Obviously the maintenance of a basement membrane is evidence of a quiescent interface between the epidermis and a specialized form of connective tissue known as the papillary dermis, with a similar relationship between other examples of cutaneous epithelia and their stroma. The papillary dermis is a specialized matrix that is comparable to the lamina propria of the digestive tract.

Invasion is manifested by extension of tumor cells into the dermis in one or more foci. Initially invasion is confined to the papillary dermis, but at this level has little or no clinical significance. Invasion is indicated by a variety of changes. The evaluation of invasion by an experienced pathologist is usually a subjective process that is difficult to verbalize.

The following histologic features are indicative of invasion.

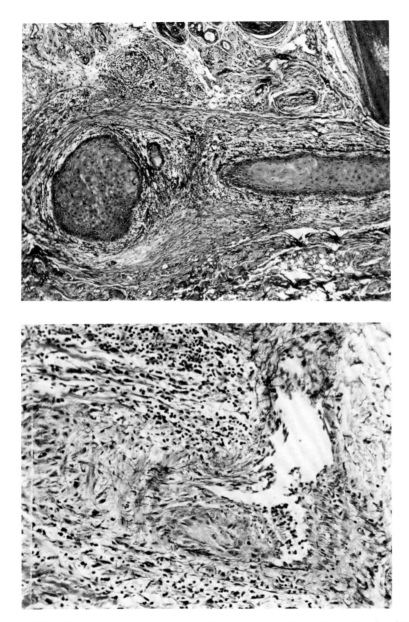

Fig. 5-23. Deep margin of keratoacanthoma (minimal keratinocytic dysplasia) showing blood vessel invasion. VVG.

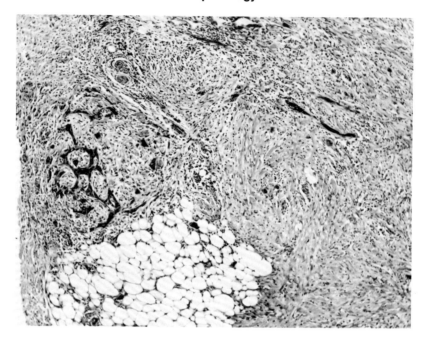

Fig. 5-24. Deep margin of keratoacanthoma showing extension of small fascicles of cells into an active fibrous stroma and into the subcutaneous fat. This is a worrisome pattern of growth when present at the advancing margin of a keratoacanthoma. (Same lesion as shown in Fig. 5-22.)

1. Extension of epithelial processes beyond normal confines.
2. Lymphohistiocytic infiltrates surrounding abnormal epithelial processes.
3. Dissolution of basement membrane.
4. Partial loss of basal cell layer surrounding abnormal cellular aggregates.
5. Isolation of nests of tumor cells in the dermis.

An evaluation of each of these features is required to confirm the presence of dermal invasion.

It is difficult to identify dermal invasion positively if the abnormal epithelium is confined to the papillary dermis. If the process has extended into the reticular dermis, then significant invasion has occurred.

Lymphohistiocytic infiltrates are present in the dermis beneath many premalignant epithelial dysplasias of the skin. They are preponderantly perivascular, but may be diffuse in the papillary dermis. They may obliterate the normal interface between epithelium and dermis. In areas where the infiltrate extends into the abnormal (clonal) epithelial process, there

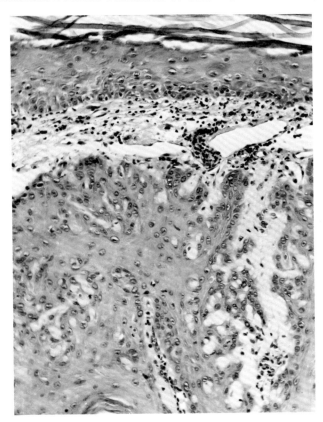

Fig. 5-25. Well-differentiated epidermoid carcinoma infiltrating the dermis beneath an epidermis that shows a minimal amount of keratinocytic dysplasia. The tumor cells, which have not stimulated a reactive stroma, are infiltrating actinically damaged connective tissue and have extruded this altered elastotic material into their interstices.

is usually destruction of its basement membrane and its basal layers (Fig. 5-26). This reactive process in which lymphohistiocytic infiltrates obliterate a dermoepithelial interface and destroy the basal epithelial layer may be characterized as lichenoid. It is the characteristic inflammatory response in lichen planus. It regularly occurs in premalignant (clonal) keratoses of the skin (Fig. 5-27). It probably is an immune response that is mediated at a cellular level. It occurs in the absence of clearcut evidence of dermal invasion. There is histologic evidence that keratinized cells are antigenic, and if present in the dermis they function as foreign bodies. Keratiniz-

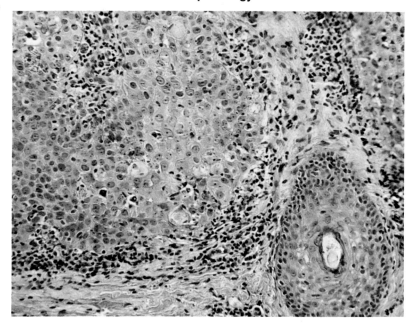

Fig. 5-26. Intermediate keratinocytic dysplasia (carcinoma in situ) showing an irregular extension of cytologically malignant cells into the papillary dermis with compression of the underlying reticular dermis. The nest of cells is surrounded by an infiltrate of lymphocytes and histiocytes that in some areas has produced a lichenoid pattern with destruction of the basal layer.

ing cells normally are "protected" from defense processes of the dermis by the basement membrane and its supportive basal epithelial cells. If clonal keratoses are recognized as "foreign" by the host, and if the recognition is indicated by lymphohistiocytic infiltrates, then it follows that either the basement membrane or its supportive basal cells are defective (they fail to isolate the keratinocytes of the intermediate layer from defense processes in the dermis).

Small nests of tumor cells that are "isolated" in the dermis are indicative of invasion. If the nests of cells show one or more areas in which basal cells are absent or are altered to resemble keratinocytes of the intermediate layer (Fig. 5-26), then the evidence for invasion is strengthened. If a nest of cells extends into the dermis but maintains an attachment to the epidermis, the evidence of true invasion requires demonstration of

1. extension into the reticular dermis,

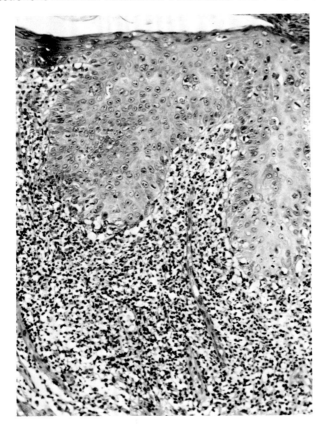

Fig. 5-27. Intermediate keratinocytic dysplasia (carcinoma in situ) showing a thickened papillary dermis that is infiltrated with lymphocytes and histiocytes. The infiltrate hugs the abnormal epithelium and produces a lichenoid pattern with the formation of colloid bodies and with focal destruction of the basal layer. Atypism is moderate in this field.

2. trapping of connective fibers of reticular dermis in interstices of epithelial cells,
3. focal loss of basement membrane,
4. focal alteration or destruction of basal layer at the periphery of the suspicious nest of cells.

Items 3 and 4 cannot be accepted as clearcut evidence of dermal invasion if the suspicious nest of cells is confined to the papillary dermis. An interplay between stroma and epithelium at the level of the papillary dermis may be accepted as within the range of normal responses of the skin to injury. This interplay at the level of the papillary dermis is characterized by epidermal hyperplasia, by attrition of epidermal cells at the dermo-epidermal interface, and by accretion of newly formed connective tissue at the surface of the papillary dermis to fill in the epidermal defects. In most examples the attrition of epidermal cells at the dermoepidermal interface is associated with an infiltrate of lymphocytes and histiocytes. The reaction has features of an immune response that is mediated at the cellular level (lichenoid reaction).

In general, the growth pattern of a tumor may be correlated with its behavior. Biologically low grade tumors are expansile, and tend to have rounded contours and to compress adjacent tissue. The common type of basal cell carcinoma with an induced stroma is a classic example of a low grade carcinoma with pushing margins (Fig. 5-6). Tumors with reactive stromas are more likely to infiltrate widely or to metastasize and are characterized by irregular extensions from the main tumor mass (Fig. 5-28).

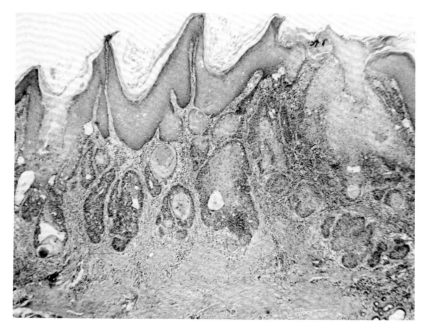

Fig. 5-28. Epidermoid carcinoma of the skin showing infiltration to about the level of the sweat glands. Some of the nests of cells show acantholysis with the formation of mucin-filled clefts (acantholytic epidermoid carcinoma; adenoacanthoma). The tumor is surrounded by an inflamed reactive stroma. The reticular dermis has been replaced by the reactive stroma in advance of the tumor.

They are more likely to be associated with blood vessel invasion and extension along peripheral nerves. Some low grade keratinocytic tumors that are expansile produce attrition of dermal connective tissue with little or no induced or reactive stroma (Fig. 5-29).

THE EVOLUTION OF CUTANEOUS CARCINOMA

In studying the evolution of human carcinomas, it is important to study variants that evolve slowly and are characterized by the stepwise acquisition of properties that equate with malignancy. As a model of human cutaneous carcinogenesis, the neoplastic system induced by actinic exposure is ideal. It provides evidence that for long periods of time some evolving neoplastic systems are characterized by an interplay at epithelial-stromal interfaces. During this period of evolution, one or more nests of

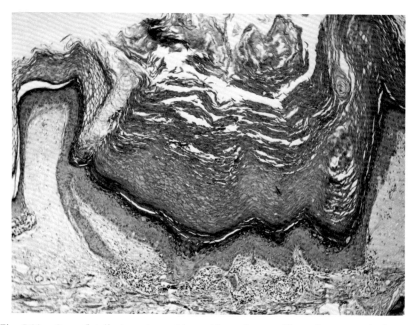

Fig. 5-29. Superficially invasive epidermoid carcinoma. There is no convincing evidence of active invasion of the dermis but the tumor cells have extended through the actinically damaged connective tissue to the level of the underlying reticular dermis to produce a cup-shaped lesion. This is a rather indolent pattern of growth in which tumor cells invade by expansion and displacement of the adjacent dermis. This expansile form of growth should be compared with the infiltrating pattern of growth seen in Fig. 5-28.

cells may transgress the basement membrane to explore the dermal connective tissue. Initially, these explorations are unsuccessful, but they result in two important reactions: (1) The unsuccessful clone of squamous cells has exposed itself to defense processes of the host. It has failed to survive the immune reaction but has altered the host. (2) The lymphocytes that respond to the exploratory thrust have recognized neoplastic squamous cells.

An interplay between recognized, neoplastic squamous cells and acquainted lymphocytes continues at the level of the basement membrane. This reciprocal interplay produces progressive and regressive changes in these two populations of cells. The squamous cells are progressively altered by the actions of the acquainted lymphocytes. The modifications in the recognized squamous cells are disguises. Each disguise in turn induces new recognition patterns in the lymphocytes. When the recognized squamous cells are successfully disguised, they may invade, proliferate, and survive in the dermis. If they invade but are incompletely disguised, they are recognized and are again partially or completely destroyed (regressive changes).

Our speculations regarding cutaneous carcinogenesis are supported by similar processes in experimental models (Foulds). They are also supported by evidence provided by recent clinicopathologic studies of human cutaneous melanoma (Clark). The radial growth phases of three clinical variants of human melanoma (superficial spreading variant, lentigo maligna, and acral lentiginous variant) are models of the interplay between evolving recognized tumor cells and the reacting, acquainted lymphocytes of the host. As Foulds has clearly indicated, and as Clark has confirmed, for each tumor in a neoplastic system that slowly evolves by the acquisition of properties that equate with malignancy, there is a similar tumor that bypasses most of the evolutionary steps to become a de novo malignancy. The variant of human cutaneous melanoma that is classified as nodular melanoma is the de novo variant of the neoplastic system of human cutaneous melanocytes. Its biologic behavior confirms its classification as a fully evolved malignancy.

The actinic or solar keratosis is an actinically induced, clonal disease of the epidermis. It is an evolutionary phase that corresponds to the radial growth phases of human cutaneous melanoma. It represents a stage in which recognized keratinocytes are evolving to progressively acquire malignant properties, and acquainted lymphocytes are progressively evolving to recognize altered keratinocytes and to acquire properties that induce regressive changes in the keratinocytes. This interplay continues until a dermal colony is established. Even at this stage, some properties that equate with malignancy may be lacking. Actinic carcinomas are common, but they rarely produce progressive local disease or metastases. Survival of tumor cells in the dermis does not equate with a fully evolved malignancy. The progressive and regressive phenomena continue after the tumor has established residency in the dermis. They may result in destruction of the dermal colony (spontaneous regression). Alternatively, they may induce progressive changes with the eventual acquisition of the properties of a fully evolved malignancy.

The de novo squamous cell carcinoma is usually a fully evolved malignant neoplasm. It arises spontaneously in undamaged skin and has a propensity for aggressive local growth and metastasis that is seldom displayed by evolved actinic carcinomas.

The second variant of premalignant keratinocytic dysplasia (intermediate keratinocytic variant) usually presents in the clinical setting of Bowen's disease. In this variant, the interplay at the dermoepidermal interface between clonal lymphocytic infiltrates and progressively evolving keratinocytes is less conspicuous than that in actinic keratosis. This observation is apparently related to a relatively intact basal layer of keratinocytes (and their basement membrane) between the intermediate dysplastic keratinocytes and the lymphoid infiltrates. In areas in which the interface is transgressed by lymphocytes, the progressive and regressive phenomena are operative. It is in these sites that evidence of early invasion is most likely to be found.

The primary actinically induced alteration that predisposes to epithelial carcinogenesis has not been clearly defined. Much of the speculation has centered around changes in dermal connective tissue and vascularity. Almost certainly the primary alteration is in keratinocytes and may be reflected in a defective basement membrane. The normal basement membrane probably represents an immunologic barrier. If antibodies to keratinocytes or if aggressive lymphocytes transgress the barrier, the membrane is defective. The initial insult to a damaged basement membrane is twofold: keratinocytes are altered and they are acquainted with lymphocytes. The latter initiate a process that favors regression of the altered keratinocytes. Unfortunately the aggressive lymphocytes may initiate changes in the keratinocytes that favor progressive rather than regressive phenomena.

There is experimental evidence that in early phases of an evolving malignancy the aggressive lymphocytes may stimulate their target cells (Prehn). If these observations are applicable to human neoplasia, we may have an explanation for the process that we recognize as keratoacanthoma. The latter tumor may represent the stimulated phase of an evolving carcinoma. It is characterized by a refractory stroma. When lymphoid infiltrates are well developed in a keratoacanthoma, there is usually evidence of focal regressive phenomena, such as focal stimulation of a reactive stroma and degeneration of infiltrating keratinocytes. Those keratoacanthomas that persist as carcinomas may be a result of the interplay between progressive and regressive phenomena. In the interplay of progressive and regressive phenomena, clones of keratinocytes may acquire the properties of malignant cells.

In discussions of the differentiation of basal cell carcinomas from other basal cell tumors such as trichoepitheliomas, emphasis is often placed on the presence of lymphohistiocytic infiltrates in carcinomas. Some well-differentiated basal cell carcinomas stimulate relatively little or no inflammation. With few or no exceptions, those basal cell carcinomas that lack an inflammatory component are characterized by induced stroma. Those that have significant components of inflammatory infiltrates are usually associated with reactive stromas.

Chapter 6

Controversies
in Dermatopathology

ATYPICAL FIBROUS XANTHOMA
AND SPINDLE CELL CARCINOMA

Presentation of the Controversy

The concept of spindle cell carcinoma of the skin, once firmly entrenched in the medical literature, is now viewed with suspicion. The poorly differentiated squamous cell carcinoma that is not keratinizing, but retains an epithelial pattern with nests of tumor cells separated by an active fibrous stroma, does not present a problem for the pathologist. The difficulty arises when a spindle cell malignant tumor of the skin assumes sarcomatoid patterns with isolation of individual tumor cells by a fibrous or myxomatous matrix (Figs. 6-1 and 6-2). To be included in this problem category, the lesion should be additionally distinguished by a close association with an epithelial surface, either the epidermis or a skin appendage such as a pilosebaceous unit. This section is primarily concerned with tumors that satisfy the following criteria.

1. They have an intimate association with an epithelial surface (usually the epidermis) (Fig. 6-3).
2. At the interface between the epithelial surface and the tumor there is partial or complete loss of the basal layer with apparent blending of keratinocytes and tumor cells (Fig. 6-4).
3. The tumor cells may be compactly arranged in one or more areas, but generally show large areas of sarcomatoid patterns in which individual cells are isolated in a fibrous matrix (Fig. 6-5).

Tumors that fulfill the above criteria fall into one of two categories. They are either diffusely infiltrating malignancies having poorly outlined margins, or they are sharply circumscribed and tend to remain confined to the dermis. Tumors satisfying the above criteria are closely associated with damaged dermal connective tissue. The injury to the dermal connective tissue usually is in the form of actinic damage, but may be the result of x-irradiation or thermal injury.

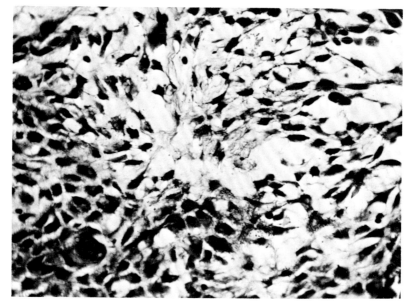

Fig. 6-1. Spindle cell carcinoma of the skin showing a zone of transition from loosely adherent keratinocytes (prickle cells) to a sarcomatoid pattern in which spindle and stellate cells are loosely arranged in a myxomatous matrix.

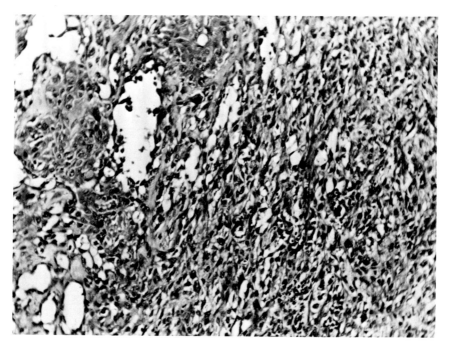

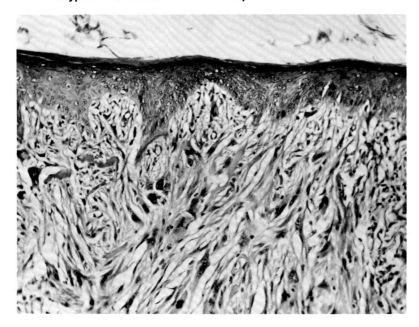

Fig. 6-3. So-called atypical fibroxanthoma showing pleomorphic spindle cells in a fibrous matrix. The tumor cells press upon the overlying epidermis and in some areas appear to blend with the basal portion of the epidermis.

Although there has been a recent trend to deny the existence of spindle cell carcinoma, the evidence against the concept is inconclusive. One of the main reasons that the concept of spindle cell carcinoma has fallen into disfavor has been the popularization of the concept of atypical fibroxanthoma (Fig. 6-6). Most of the lesions classified as atypical fibroxanthoma would also satisfy the criteria listed above for spindle cell carcinoma. These lesions are additionally characterized by an expansile pattern of growth and almost invariably are confined to the dermis. They are distinguished also by regional variation in pattern with scattered areas showing evidence of maturation, such as reduction in cellularity, decreased cellular atypism, and increased prominence of intercellular matrix.

Fig. 6-2. Sarcomatoid tumor of the skin of an elderly patient with actinic damage showing a zone of transition from acantholytic epidermoid carcinoma to a sarcomatoid pattern in which spindle cells are isolated in a fibrous matrix. In some areas the histologic pattern is indistinguishable from that seen in so-called atypical fibroxanthoma. The tumor is distinguished by the presence of recognizable squamous cell carcinoma and by demonstrable transitions from the squamous cell carcinoma to the sarcomatoid pattern.

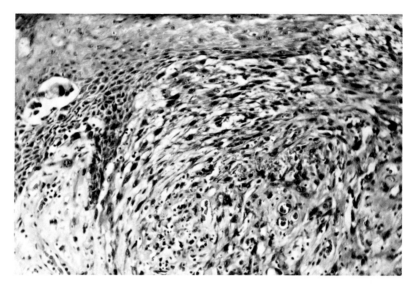

Fig. 6-4. Recurrent atypical fibroxanthoma showing an area of keratinocytic dysplasia with acantholysis at the left-hand margin of the field. Atypical fibroblastic spindle cells have concentrated at the interface between the epidermis and the underlying tumor and appear to blend with the zone of keratinocytic dysplasia on the left.

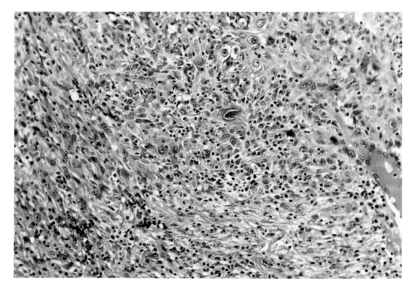

Fig. 6-5. In this atypical fibroxanthoma there is a zone of transition from keratinocytes to fibroblastic spindle cells.

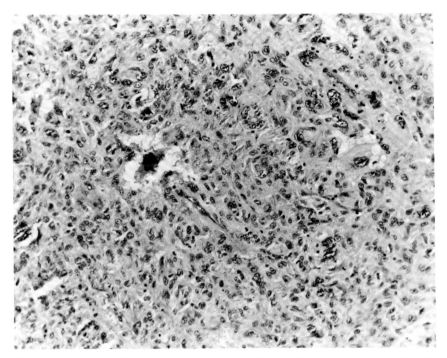

Fig. 6-6. Atypical fibroxanthoma showing a characteristic pattern of epithelioid cells, fibroblastic spindle cells, and tumor giant cells.

Most tumors selected on the basis of the criteria outlined above (sarcomatoid patterns, continuity with epithelial surface, and damaged skin) will behave in a relatively benign fashion. They may occasionally recur locally but seldom metastasize. Within the group of tumors that do metastasize, a review of the histologic section will almost invariably show that the lesion was uniformly cellular and had an infiltrating pattern of growth extending beyond the confines of the dermis.

One additional feature that is sometimes emphasized in the diagnosis of spindle cell carcinoma is the presence of nests of keratinizing squamous epithelium within the tumor. These nests usually show one or more areas in which the basal layer is absent, or they occasionally may show areas in which the basal layer shows loss of cohesion and blends with tumor cells in the fibrous stroma (Fig. 6-7). This lack of cohesion between basal cells and keratinizing squamous cells is a feature of a special subcategory of squamous cell carcinoma of the skin (adenoacanthoma; acantholytic epidermoid carcinoma) (Fig. 6-8). Occasionally keratinocytic dysplasia with evidence of acantholysis between the basal layer and the overlying

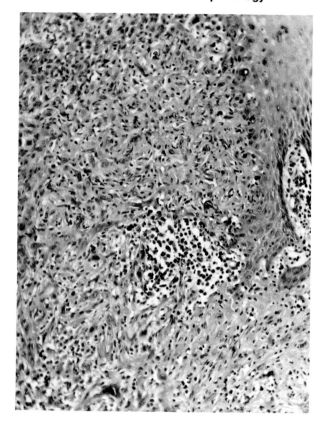

Fig. 6-7. In this atypical fibroxanthoma there is a transition from acantholytic squamous epithelium to fibroblastic spindle cells. Inflammatory cells have clustered in the acantholytic clefts in the keratinocytic portion of the tumor.

keratinocytes is present in the epidermis bordering an otherwise characteristic atypical fibroxanthoma (Fig. 6-9).

If the histology of atypical fibroxanthoma is ignored, there are remarkable similarities between its growth pattern and biologic behavior and those of actinic squamous cell carcinoma of the skin. There is a good deal of indirect evidence to support the concept that most of the lesions classified as atypical fibroxanthomas may actually be squamous cell carcinomas that have converted to a sarcomatoid pattern. For this group of lesions we will use the term transformed carcinomas. The association between acantholytic epidermoid carcinoma and transformed carcinomas (atypical fibroxanthomas) may be evidence that the former is the direct precursor of the latter. Often the clefts formed in a nest of acantholytic

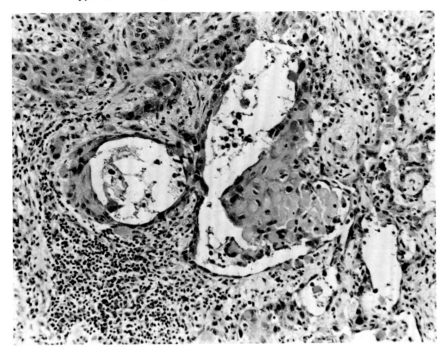

Fig. 6-8. Acantholytic epidermoid carcinoma showing mucin-filled clefts containing an infiltrate of chronic inflammatory cells. Many of the acantholytic cells also show dyskeratosis. The tumor cells are embedded in a reactive stroma containing infiltrates of chronic inflammatory cells. This acantholytic epidermoid carcinoma was located approximately 1 cm from an atypical fibroxanthoma. Keratinocytic dysplasia was present in the epidermis between these two lesions.

epidermoid carcinoma contain a stringy mucinous matrix (Fig. 6-8). Although this matrix has been accepted as evidence of glandular differentiation (adenoacanthomas) it may actually be evidence of mesenchymal metaplasia with conversion of basal cells to cells that are potential fibrocytes.

The evidence that atypical fibroxanthomas are histiocytic tumors is based upon the following observations.

1. Many of the cells have epithelioid characteristics.
2. Stromal hemorrhages with hemosiderin deposits are prominent.
3. Xanthoma cells may be present but are not a striking feature of most atypical fibroxanthomas.
4. There is often an admixture of spindle and epithelioid cells that super-

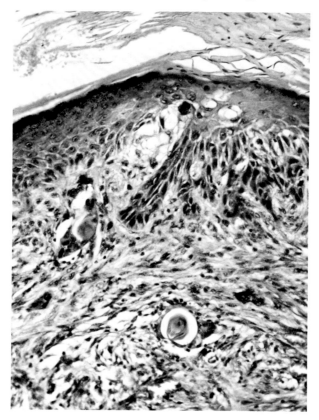

Fig. 6-9. In this atypical fibroxanthoma, fibroblastic tumor cells appear to blend with altered keratinocytes. Keratinocytic dysplasia is evident in the adjacent epidermis.

ficially resembles the fibrocytes and histiocytes of lesions in the fibro-xanthoma group.

5. Lesions that are otherwise typical fibroxanthomas of the skin (dermato-fibromas) may show regional variation in pattern with nuclear pleo-morphism and anaplasia.

There is a resemblance between transformed carcinomas (atypical fibro-xanthomas) and lesions in category 5. For lesions in the latter category we use the term atypical dermatofibroma. This type of lesion is often sharply circumscribed and may not show the characteristic loose infiltration at lateral margins seen in the usual example of dermatofibroma. The component cells tend to be rather plump and show varying degrees of nuclear atypism. There is regional variation in pattern and occasionally there are areas containing numerous bizarre multinucleated cells. Some of these cells have characteristics of touton type of giant cells and contain fine cytoplasmic vacuoles. Many of the mononuclear cells have histiocytic characteristics and some of these contain cytoplasmic vacuoles of the type associated with storage of lipids. The vascular pattern is often well developed and occasionally is sinusoidal. The tumor usually spares the upper portion of the dermis. The close association between epidermis and tumor that is characteristic of atypical fibroxanthoma is usually not a feature of the atypical dermatofibroma, which is additionally distinguished by a lack of an association with damage to dermal connective tissue and by a preference for a younger age group (usually less than 30 years of age).

The pathologist is usually hesitant to assign to the category of atypical fibroxanthoma tumors that satisfy the criteria listed above for transformed carcinoma but infiltrate at their deep margin to extend along peripheral nerves and beyond the confines of the dermis. Such lesions present a problem in classification. They may be assigned to the category of spindle cell carcinoma without any real assurance that such a lesion exists.

The Sarcomatoid Transformation of Carcinomas

If some or all of the so-called atypical fibroxanthomas of the skin are sarcomatoid or transformed carcinomas, what processes are operative in the transformation? The following are regularly observed in atypical fibroxanthomas and may be significant.

1. Varying degrees of keratinocytic dysplasia are common in the epidermis bordering an atypical fibroxanthoma.
2. Acantholysis with the formation of mucin filled clefts is characteristic of the keratinocytic dysplasia.
3. Nests of dysplastic acantholytic keratinocytes are occasionally present in atypical fibroxanthomas.
4. These keratinocytic dysplasias are of the basal cell or actinic type.
5. In areas where the sarcomatoid portion is in contact with the epidermis, the basal keratinocytic layer is usually absent.
6. In areas in which a transition from dysplastic keratinocytes to sarcomatoid spindle cells can be demonstrated, the interstices of the transforming keratinocytes are widened and contain an infiltrate of lymphocytes and histiocytes.

The acantholytic basal cell pattern of keratinocytic dysplasia is seen with sufficient regularity in transformed carcinomas of the skin to be accepted as a pattern of dysplasia that predisposes to sarcomatoid transformation (Fig. 6-2). The reason for this proclivity in acantholytic basal cell dysplasia is uncertain but may be related to the mucinous matrix that fills the widened interstitial spaces. It is reasonable to assume that this mucinous matrix is a product of the dysplastic keratinocyte. The other commonly observed feature in carcinomas that show sarcomatoid transformation is infiltration of the widened mucin-filled interstitial spaces by lymphocytes and histiocytes (Fig. 6-10). It is tempting to speculate that the sarcomatoid transformation of acantholytic dysplastic keratinocytes is mediated by the lymphohistiocytic infiltrate. The histiocytes may assume fibrocytic properties and convert the epithelial interstitium to a fibrous matrix. As a result the neoplastic keratinocytes are isolated from their neighbors by the histiocytic mediated stroma and assume sarcomatoid characteristics. This transformation would appear to involve primarily the dysplastic basal layer, which loses its identity in zones of transition. The basal keratinocyte is a specialized cell that bridges the gap between dermis on one side and maturing keratinocyte on the opposite side. Although there is no evidence that the basal keratinocyte is fibrogenic, it does play a role in formation of the basal lamina. The basal lamina func-

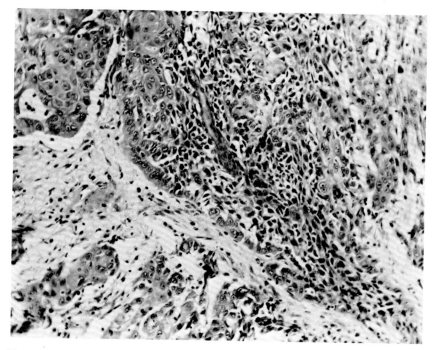

Fig. 6-10. Acantholytic epidermoid carcinoma showing spindle cell transformation with an infiltrate of inflammatory cells in the zone of transformation.

tions as a site of epidermal attachment but may also be an immunologic barrier. Since the basal keratinocyte can function and survive in contact with dermal collagen, it may be classified as a facultative dermatocyte.

"NEUROID" SPINDLE CELL TUMORS

Within the category of spindle cell neoplasms that arise in damaged dermis is a distinctive tumor that is distinguished by its behavior and by its fasciculation and neurotropism. The histogenesis of this variant is uncertain but it probably corresponds to some of the lesions which have been classified as desmoplastic melanoma. The lesions we have included in this section are amelanotic. Their origin from epidermal melanocytes is unproved. The tumor cells blend with the basal portion of the epidermis, forming elongated fascicles that infiltrate the dermis and underlying soft tissue (Fig. 6-11). The fascicles blend with peripheral nerves. They infiltrate the perineurium and endoneurium. They radiate from the infiltrated nerves in a pattern reminiscent of that seen in traumatic neuromas (Fig.

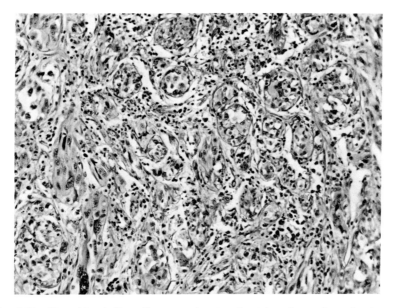

Fig. 6-11. Neuroid spindle cell tumor showing fascicles of spindle cells that are clearly outlined by fibrous membranes. The fascicles are tortuous and are cut in longitudinal and cross section. The pattern is reminiscent of that seen in traumatic neuromas.

6-12). The fascicles of tumor cells are additionally distinguished by reticulin fibers, which outline the fascicles and many of the individual tumor cells. The fibers are also PAS positive and have characteristics of basement membranes. The fibers, which are relatively straight and rigid, are similar to those produced by schwann cells. Argyrophilic fibers are also demonstrated in the fascicles of tumor cells with Bodian's stain. It is not certain whether these are neurites, which accompany the tumor cells, or neuroglia fibers.

These spindle cell malignancies are distinguished by their fasciculated pattern, their reticulum pattern, their neurotropism, and their absence of pigment production. They are associated with keratinocytic and melanocytic dysplasias, but it is difficult to identify a cell of origin in the epidermis. The tumor cells have schwann cell characteristics. If they are of melanocytic origin, they are comparable to neurotized nevus cells. These lesions might be classified as neurotized melanomas or as primary malignant schwannomas.

Clinicopathologic Correlation

This tumor is characterized by repeated local recurrences with progressive extension along peripheral nerves. There is often evidence of progres-

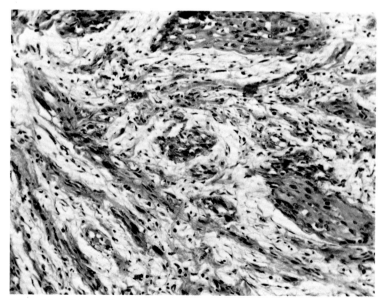

Fig. 6-12. Neuroid spindle cell tumor showing parallel fascicles of tumor cells in a loose fibrous matrix.

sive dedifferentiation with more pronounced degrees of nuclear atypism in the recurrences. The tumor may eventually extend into the cranial cavity or may produce lymphatic or blood-borne metastases.

CUTANEOUS MALIGNANT MELANOMA

The surgical pathology of cutaneous neoplasms requires special techniques to demonstrate patterns of growth, depth of invasion, and routes of spread. In addition, microscopic interpretations are concerned with dysplastic precursors, tumor grades (degrees of differentiation), patterns of infiltration, and host responses. Finally, clinicopathologic correlations may significantly influence therapeutic decisions. Many of these aspects of the surgical pathology of the skin are exemplified by a study of malignant melanomas.

The classification of cutaneous malignant melanomas has evolved from clinicopathologic correlations. Malignant melanomas of the skin are usually classified in one of the following three categories:

1. nodular
2. superficial spreading
3. lentigo maligna

Occasionally it is impossible to categorize a cutaneous melanoma in one of these groups. Melanomas of the palms and soles are often exceptions and have distinctive histologic features (lentiginous acral melanomas).

Nodular or De Novo Melanoma

The nodular or de novo malignant melanoma is invasive almost from its inception. If lateral growth of tumor cells in the epidermis occurs, it is rapidly followed by extensions of tumor into the dermis. As a result, lateral intraepithelial growth is rarely evident at a distance greater than two rete ridges from a site of dermal invasion. De novo malignant melanomas tend to transgress the papillary dermis rapidly to invade the reticular dermis. Their interface with the reticular dermis is often obscured by lymphohistiocytic infiltrates (reactive stroma), but in some examples or as a regional variation in pattern, they extend between collagen bundles with little or no inflammatory reaction (refractory stroma). Melanomas with reactive stromas usually grow in an expansile fashion with pushing margins. Collagen bundles of the reticular dermis are resorbed by the reactive stroma in advance of the tumor cells. Melanomas with refractory stromas grow in an infiltrating fashion. Collagen bundles of the reticular dermis are trapped between and disrupted by the advancing tumor cells.

Superficial Spreading Malignant Melanoma

The superficial spreading malignant melanoma is characterized by a prolonged period of lateral growth at a superficial level in the skin. The tumor cells are relatively uniform, aggregate in theques in the epidermis, and, as single cells, invade all levels of the epidermis (Fig. 6-13). Dermal invasion is common and is almost invariably found if a careful search is made (Fig. 6-14). Lymphohistiocytic infiltrates border the proliferating tumor cells. The inflammatory infiltrates are evidence of host's resistance to the proliferating tumor cells. In its period of lateral growth this tumor is confined to the epidermis and the papillary dermis. During this period there is an interplay between the tumor cells and defense processes of the host. The confinement of the tumor to the epidermis and the papillary

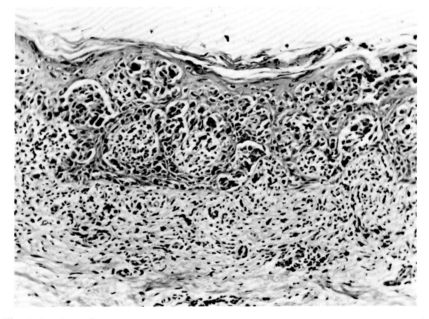

Fig. 6-13. Superficial spreading malignant melanoma showing a pagetoid pattern of epidermal invasion by atypical melanocytes. The atypical melanocytes have also aggregated near the dermoepidermal interface to form irregular theques. The papillary dermis is thickened, shows active fibroplasia, and contains a perivascular infiltrate of lymphocytes and histiocytes. There is no evidence of dermal invasion in this field (Level I growth).

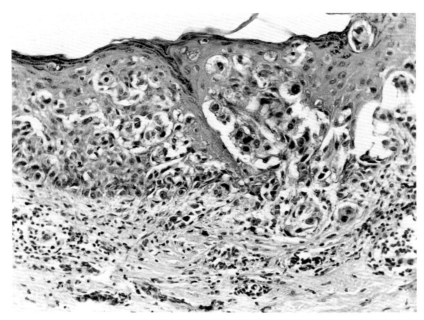

Fig. 6-14. Superficial spreading malignant melanoma showing pagetoid invasion of epidermis. The epidermis is thickened and shows an increased prominence of the granular layer. The papillary dermis shows active fibroplasia and in some areas contains nests of atypical melanocytes (Level II invasion). Infiltrates of inflammatory cells are present in the thickened papillary dermis.

dermis is evidence that the period of lateral growth is an expression of immunologic competence. In one or more sites the tumor cells may be destroyed (spontaneous involution). Eventually, either as an expression of a failure of immune processes or by an acquisition of new biologic properties by the tumor cells, the tumor extends beyond the confines of the papillary dermis to invade the reticular dermis (vertical growth phase). In the vertical growth phase the tumor assumes the biologic properties of de novo melanoma. It is distinguished from the latter by remnants of the lateral growth phase (intraepithelial growth at a distance greater than 2 or 3 rete ridges away from the main tumor mass).

Lentigo Maligna

Lentigo maligna shares with superficial spreading malignant melanoma the feature of a prolonged phase of lateral growth. It is distinguished by diffuse melanocytic hyperplasia in the epidermis (a lentiginous pattern), by an association with actinically damaged dermal connective tissue, and by cellular pleomorphism (Fig. 6-15). The neoplastic melanocytes do not invade all levels of the epidermis extensively, but tend to remain at the interface between the epidermis and the dermis. The intraepithelial growth of tumor cells extends along the outer sheath of hair follicles and along sweat ducts (Fig. 6-16). The host's response to the abnormal clone or clones of melanocytes is similar to that seen in superficial spreading malignant melanoma. Areas of spontaneous involution are common. The vertical growth phase of lentigo maligna is often multifocal. The infiltrating cells are often spindle shaped (Figs. 6-17 & 18). Lentigo maligna is additionally characterized by a relatively good prognosis even in its vertical growth phase (lentigo maligna melanoma).

There is increasing evidence that the level of dermal invasion by a malignant melanoma may be closely correlated with prognosis and survival. The levels of invasion are: Level II, loose infiltration of papillary dermis

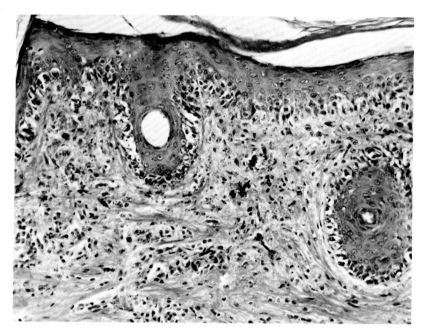

Fig. 6-15. Lentigo maligna showing diffuse atypical melanocytic hyperplasia in the basal portion of the epidermis. There is relatively little invasion of the overlying epidermis. The epidermis shows effacement of rete ridges. The granular layer is prominent and the horny layer is compact and thickened. The atypical melanocytes have extended along the outer sheath of hair follicles. The papillary dermis is thickened and shows chronic inflammation with accumulations of pigment in melanophages.

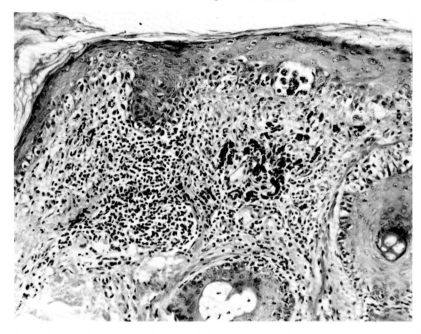

Fig. 6-16. Lentigo maligna showing diffuse atypical melanocytic hyperplasia in the basal portion of the epidermis with effacement of rete ridges. The atypical melanocytes have extended along the outer sheath of hair follicles. The papillary dermis is thickened and contains infiltrates of chronic inflammatory cells and collections of melanophages.

(Fig. 6-14) ; Level III, compact aggregates of tumor cells filling the papillary dermis and extending to interface between the papillary and reticular dermis (Fig. 6-19) ; polypoid Level III, confined to papillary dermis but polypoid at surface and compresses reticular dermis (Fig. 6-20) ; Level IV, extension into reticular dermis (Fig. 6-21) ; and Level V, invasion of the panniculus adiposus. The prognosis for tumors at Level II is excellent and is almost as good for Level III. The prognosis rapidly worsens at Level IV and is poor for tumors at Level V. Level I growth refers to tumors that are confined to the epidermis (melanoma in situ) (Fig. 6-22). There are serious objections to the clinical concept of melanoma in situ. Insurance carriers have not accepted a "benign" form of melanoma. If the tumor cells are cytologically malignant, form theques, and are confined to the epidermis, the lesion is often characterized as *active junctional nevus*. If the melanocytes show a lentiginous pattern of growth, are cytologically malignant, and are confined to the epidermis, the process is classified as lentigo maligna. W. H. Clark, Jr. has proposed a cytologic classification of atypical

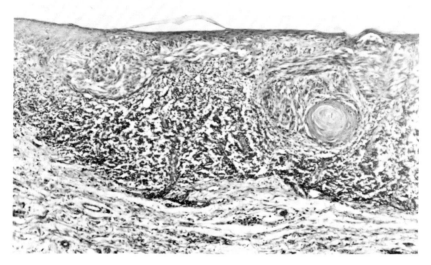

Fig. 6-17. Lentigo maligna melanoma showing irregular extensions of atypical melanocytes into a thickened inflamed papillary dermis (Level II invasion).

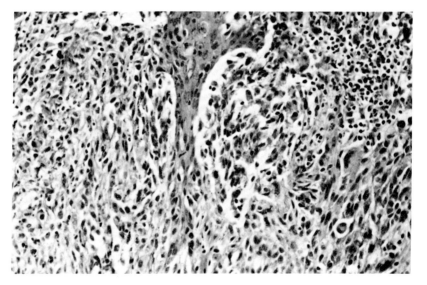

Fig. 6-18. Lentigo maligna melanoma showing nests of atypical spindle cells originating from the epidermis and infiltrating the dermis. The tumor cells show a minimal degree of dysplasia and many of the cells have features that are comparable to those seen in type A spindle cell melanomas of the eye. This spindle cell pattern is common in lentigo maligna melanoma.

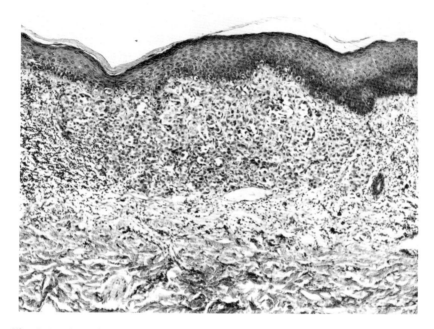

Fig. 6-19. Superficial spreading malignant melanoma showing a nodular accumulation of atypical melanocytes in a thickened papillary dermis. The nests of cells are closely aggregated and have displaced their stroma. The tumor cells have completely filled the thickened papillary dermis. In this area the lesion qualifies as Level III invasion. This tumor metastasized to regional lymph nodes.

melanocytic processes expressed in terms of degrees of dysplasia. As an alternative to the inaccurate term active junctional nevus, he proposes that such a process be classified as *marked melanocytic dysplasia*. At a practical level, dysplastic melanocytic tumors other than lentigo maligna are seldom in situ. If a sufficient number of sections are examined, it is usually possible to demonstrate one or more sites of dermal invasion.

By definition de novo melanomas are never in situ and are unlikely to be confined to Level II invasion. They may be confined to Level III invasion and, at this level, may pose serious therapeutic decisions. There are at least two categories of tumor aggregates that have been classified as Level III invasion. One category is characterized by a plaque of tumor cells with little or no elevation at the surface of the skin. Lesions in this category have a predictably good prognosis. The second category is characterized by a polypoid tumor that projects above the skin surface and appears to sit on the reticular dermis. Tumors in this category (polypoid Level III) have unpredictable behavior. Their prognosis approaches that of tumors

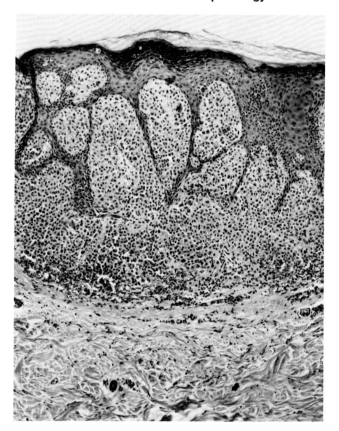

Fig. 6-20. Superficial spreading malignant melanoma with a localized area of Level III invasion. The tumor has compressed its stroma in advance of the tumor cells and is growing in an expansile fashion. The expanding tumor has compressed the reticular dermis and has produced a concave interface between the tumor and the dermis.

with Level IV invasion and we prefer to include these polypoid variants in the latter category (biologic rather than histologic classification).

The distinction between Level III invasion and Level IV invasion may be difficult to define. The elastica of the reticular dermis has different tinctorial qualities from that of the papillary dermis. The single most distinctive quality of the elastica of the reticular dermis is its PTAH positivity. If PTAH positive elastica is demonstrated in a melanoma, Level IV invasion is proved. Unfortunately the inflammatory interface of an infiltrating melanoma tends to destroy the elastica in advance of the tumor. The configuration of the interface between a "pushing" melanoma and the

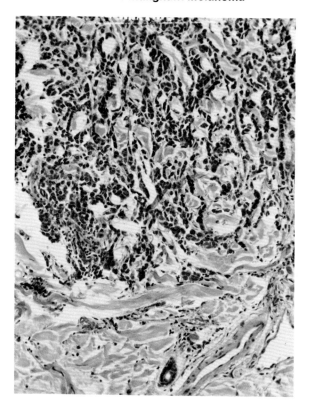

Fig. 6-21. Deep margin of malignant melanoma showing infiltrating pattern of growth. Cords of tumor cells extend between collagen bundles of the reticular dermis.

reticular dermis is important in evaluating level of invasion. If the interface on the dermal side is markedly concave, the tumor probably has a prognosis that approaches that of an infiltrating tumor that has invaded to Level IV.

The therapeutic implications of levels of invasion have not been clearly defined. There is convincing evidence that the likelihood of metastasis from tumors confined to Level II does not justify radical therapy.

Melanomas have histologic features that are indicative of the common heritage with the parent cell that gives origin to cellular nevi. With few exceptions, a melanoma differs from a cellular nevus in the relationship between tumor cells and stroma. Melanoma cells are arranged in nests and fascicles with little or no intervening stroma. The lack of respect that melanoma cells have for their stroma is evidence of an aggressive pattern

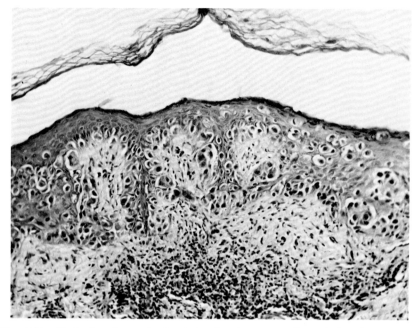

Fig. 6-22. Marked melanocytic dysplasia showing nests of atypical melanocytes at the interface between the epidermis and the dermis. Infiltration of the epidermis produces a pagetoid pattern. The papillary dermis is thickened and contains inflammatory infiltrates. (Level I growth).

of growth. Occasionally melanomas may show evidence of differentiation in one or more areas. In these areas the cells are small (nevuslike) (Fig. 6-23) and may be loosely aggregated in nests and fascicles in a fibrous stroma. This histologic pattern is difficult to distinguish from that seen in a cellular nevus. In melanomas showing these features it is difficult or impossible to be certain whether the nevuslike areas are evidence of differentiation or of the origin of the melanoma in a preexisting benign nevus (Figs. 6-24, 6-25). Nevuslike patterns are common in vertical growth phases of superficial spreading melanoma and in lentigo maligna melanoma. In some melanomas the nevus cell pattern is preponderant. Monoclonal melanomas that show nevus cell patterns may be characterized as minimal deviation variants. Such melanomas may metastasize (Figs. 6-26, 6-27, 6-28).

   In summary, the histologic features that are important in evaluating a melanocytic lesion are:

1. cytology—variation in size and staining qualities of nuclei
2. extension of atypical cells into dermis
3. relationships between stroma and tumor cells

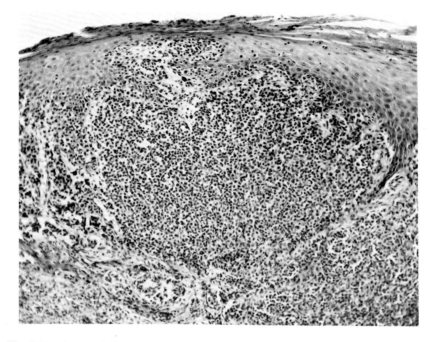

Fig. 6-23. Minimal deviation melanoma showing a nodular accumulation of small atypical cells that have nevus cell characteristics. The compression of the stroma and the relative absence of an alveolated pattern in this area are features favoring the diagnosis of minimal deviation melanoma rather than benign cellular nevus.

    a. lymphoid stroma
    b. differentiation
 4. depth of invasion
 5. presence or absence and character of lateral growth phase
 6. actinic damage
 7. vascular invasion
 8. size of tumor
 9. location of tumor
10. mitotic rate

    The proper evaluation of these features requires close correlation between the gross and microscopic findings. The gross dissection of a surgically excised melanoma requires adequate sampling of tumor nodules (vertical growth phase) and pigmented macular areas (radial growth phase), and adequate representation of margins of excision. A common source of error faced by the consultant in pathology is inadequate representation of the gross findings on the histologic preparations. For some

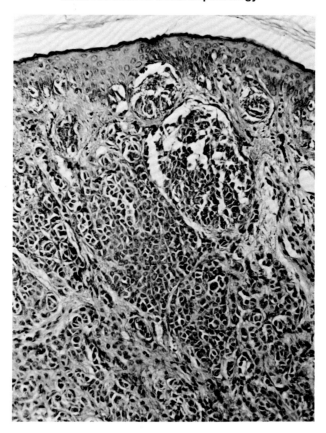

Fig. 6-24. Minimal deviation melanoma showing some irregularity in nuclear size and staining. The tumor cells are arranged in alveoli and fascicles in a delicate fibrous matrix. The arrangement of the cells mimics that seen in benign nevi. The tumor metastasized to regional lymph nodes (see also Figs. 6-26, 6-27, and 6-28).

reason, the radial growth phases are often better represented than the vertical growth phases. An erroneous prognostic evaluation may result from the interpretation of histologic sections that are not complete representations of the gross characteristics. Punch biopsies of melanomas will seldom provide adequate representation of histologic variables.

The lymphohistiocytic infiltrates that are found in the dermis beneath melanomas are expressions of the host's response to abnormal clones of melanocytes. They are regularly present in the papillary dermis in lesions of superficial spreading melanoma and in lentigo maligna. The lateral and vertical growth phases are the result of an interplay between the host's

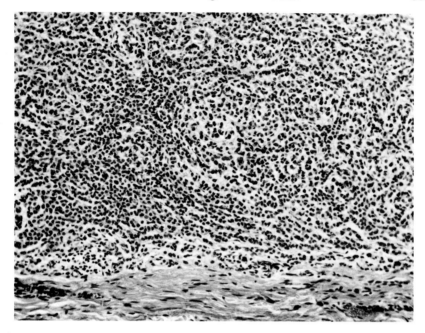

Fig. 6-25. Minimal deviation melanoma in which atypical nevuslike cells are loosely arranged in a delicate fibrous matrix. The tumor presents a uniform interface with and has compressed the reticular dermis.

resistance (lymphohistiocytic infiltrates) and the biologic aggressiveness of the tumor cells. Similar lymphohistiocytic infiltrates may be seen in halo nevi (Figs. 6-29, 6-30). They isolate, and are associated with degenerative changes in individual nevus cells. The end result of this inflammatory reaction in halo nevi is partial or complete destruction of the nevus. The implication of this destruction of a nevus is that the inflammation is the expression of an immune response. Clinically lesions of this type are often surrounded by a depigmented halo. Scattered aggregates of nevus cells with uniformly hyperchromatic nuclei are often present in either the junctional or the dermal component of a halo nevus. This nuclear atypism may be secondary to the inflammatory changes. It is tempting to propose that the nuclear changes are a morphologic expression of a primary alteration in nevus cells and are evidence of an abnormal clone (melanocytic dysplasia). The inflammation may be an expression of the host's response to such a clone of abnormal (dysplastic) nevus cells.

The histologic distinction between superficial spreading melanomas (confined to Level II) and lentigo maligna melanomas (confined to Level II) is often difficult, especially on small biopsy specimens. Lentigo ma-

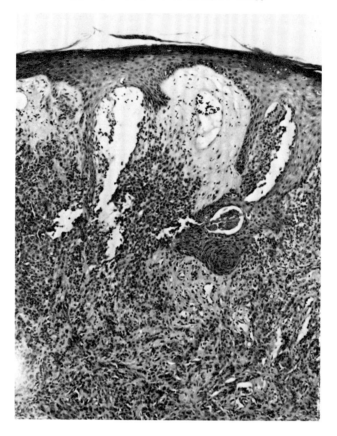

Fig. 6-26. Minimal deviation melanoma showing features of nevus cell differentiation but distinguished by slight to moderate degrees of melanocytic dysplasia. Mitoses are present.

ligna is characterized by slight to moderate atrophy of the stratum malpighii, lichenoid epidermal patterns (loss of basal layer, and hypertrophy and premature keratinization of individual keratinocytes), and diffuse hyperplasia of atypical melanocytes. The rete ridges are often effaced. The atypical melanocytes tend to remain confined to the basal portions of the epidermis. They often have well-developed dendritic processes that are distributed between keratinocytes. The melanocytic dysplasia is also characterized by anaplasia. Following fixation the atypical melanocytes tend to shrink and appear to lie within lacunae. Theques may be present and often are composed of plump atypical spindle-shaped melanocytes. Extension of the melanocytic hyperplasia along the skin appendages (hair

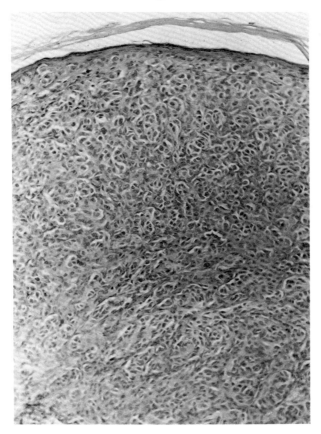

Fig. 6-27. Minimal deviation melanoma showing compactly arranged fascicles and alveoli of slightly atypical melanocytes. Mitoses are present. (Same lesion as illustrated in Figs. 6-24, 6-26, and 6-28.)

follicles and sweat ducts) is a common feature. Actinically damaged connective tissue is usually present in the reticular dermis. Lentigo maligna melanoma (Level II invasion or deeper) is often a spindle cell tumor.

Superficial spreading melanomas are primarily junctional rather than lentiginous processes. Cytologically the atypical melanocytes are relatively uniform. There may be lentiginous hyperplasia of melanocytes in the basal portion of the epidermis, but this feature is usually accompanied by single cell infiltration of the overlying epidermis to produce a pagetoid pattern and by the aggregation of cells in rounded nests. The epidermis is usually acanthotic and shows regular elongation of rete ridges especially in areas showing pagetoid patterns of infiltration. The melanocytes are

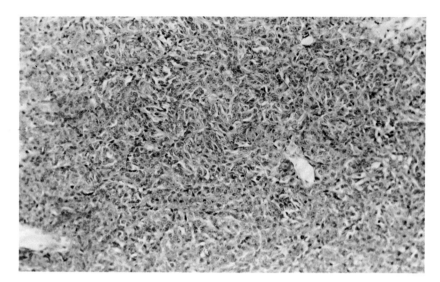

Fig. 6-28. Minimal deviation melanoma metastatic to lymph node. The tumor is cytologically similar to the primary lesion. (Figs. 6-24, 6-26, and 6-27.)

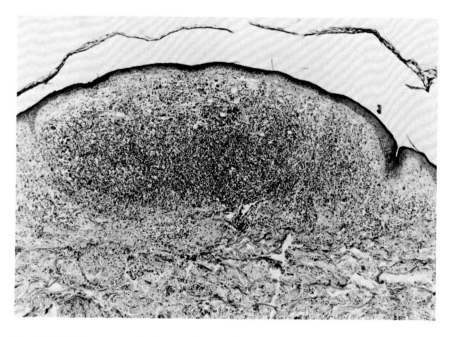

Fig. 6-29. Halo nevus showing nodular infiltrate of lymphocytes in upper portion of the dermis. The epidermis shows effacement of rete ridges. Large epithelioid cells (nevus cells) with hyperchromatic nuclei are present in the infiltrate.

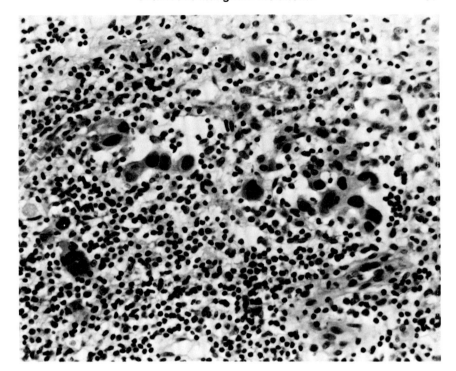

Fig. 6-30. Higher magnification of tumor shown in Fig. 6-29. The nevus cells have an abundant amount of cytoplasm and irregular uniformly hyperchromatic nuclei. They are loosely arranged in a lymphoid stroma.

usually epithelioid rather than spindle shaped. They are in close apposition to adjacent tumor cells and keratinocytes and seldom show the shrinkage artifact that characterizes the melanocytes in lentigo maligna. Dendritic processes may be inconspicuous or may form a tangle between tumor cells in the theques. Extension of the atypical melanocytes along the skin appendages is not a common feature. Occasionally a clear-cut histologic distinction between lentigo maligna and superficial spreading melanoma cannot be made.

Acral Lentiginous Melanoma

The currently popular classifications of malignant melanoma do not give recognition to a variant that with rare exceptions originates on palmar or plantar surfaces. For this group of lesions we use the term acral lentiginous melanoma. These lesions are characterized by marked acanthosis, elongation of rete ridges, and lentiginous proliferation of atypical melanocytes in the epidermis (Fig. 6-31). The lesion has a significant lateral growth phase to produce a large pigmented halo. There is usually evidence of dermal invasion in one or more areas. The tumor cells in the dermis are often spindle shaped and are arranged in fascicles. In many areas they have nevus cell characteristics with individual cells surrounded by a delicately fibrous matrix. In some of the fibrosing areas the pattern resembles that seen in blue nevi. This pattern of melanoma is histologically deceptive and may be easily misdiagnosed on small biopsies. Some of the acral melanomas are desmoplastic (Figs. 6-32, 6-33).

Definition of Levels of Invasion

Level I growth refers to those lesions in which the abnormal melanocytes are confined to the epidermis. This is the example of pure centrifugal or radial growth. Level II invasion refers to processes in which there is radial

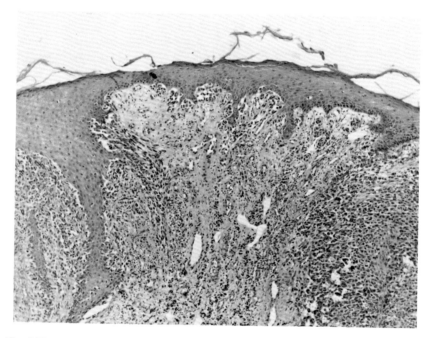

Fig. 6-31. Acral lentiginous melanoma (plantar surface) showing lentiginous pattern of atypical melanocytes at dermoepidermal interface. Fascicles of spindle-shaped tumor cells extend into a dense fibrous matrix. This type of stromal response is common in acral melanomas and may be related in part to the repeated trauma in a weight-bearing area.

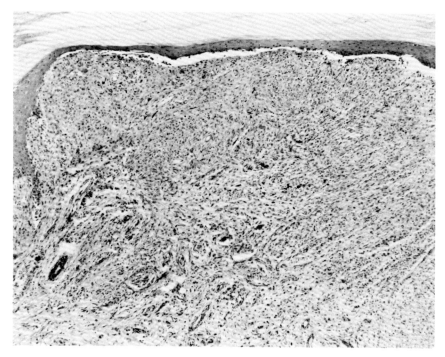

Fig. 6-32. Desmoplastic malignant melanoma showing isolation of individual tumor cells in a fibrous matrix. This is a common pattern of differentiation in the invasive portions of an acral lentiginous melanoma.

growth with widely distributed exploratory thrusts into the papillary dermis. These exploratory thrusts are characterized by one or more foci in which single neoplastic cells or scattered nests of neoplastic cells are loosely arranged in a thickened papillary dermis. Level III invasion (initial vertical growth) refers to tumors in which there are compact aggregates of neoplastic cells in a slightly to moderately thickened papillary dermis. The aggregated cells completely fill the papillary dermis and press upon the reticular dermis or upon a reactive stroma that separates the reticular dermis from the tumor cells. At low magnification the surface of the reticular dermis may be relatively straight from one margin to the opposite margin of the tumor, or it may be compressed (concave surface). Level IV invasion refers to tumors that have infiltrated the reticular dermis. If the tumor is infiltrating the dermis without stimulating a reactive stroma, it is easily recognized as Level IV invasion. If the tumor is growing in a pushing expansile fashion, the interface between tumor and reticular dermis may be obscured by a reactive stroma (Fig. 6-19 and 6-20). In such an

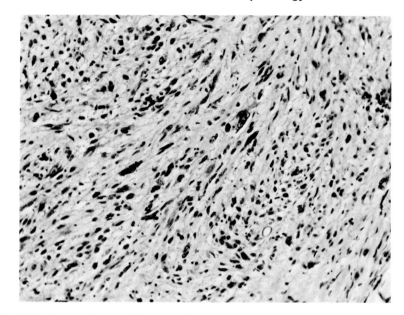

Fig. 6-33. Desmoplastic malignant melanoma showing atypical spindle cells that are loosely arranged in a fibrous matrix. Isolation of tumor cells in a fibrous matrix produces a sarcomatoid pattern and qualifies the tumor as desmoplastic. (Same tumor as illustrated in Fig. 6-32.)

example the tumor is best evaluated under low magnification. Tumors that are polypoid and compress the reticular dermis histologically are polypoid Level III lesions but biologically behave as Level IV lesions. Level V invasion refers to extension into the subcutaneous fat and is usually not a problem in microscopic evaluation.

Interpretation of Histologic Patterns and Correlation with Levels of Invasion

Two of the three accepted variants of malignant melanoma, lentigo maligna and superficial spreading melanoma, are distinguished by a prolonged period of progressive radial spread in the epidermis and the papillary dermis. The implication of this peculiar pattern of growth is that abnormal melanocytes in the epidermis are relatively protected from immune processes. The basement membrane may function as a barrier to cellularly mediated immune processes. Where this barrier is breached, the immune processes may destroy the abnormal clones of cells to produce partial or complete spontaneous regression. Abnormal melanocytes are repeatedly fed from the intraepidermal clone into the papillary dermis. In the early phases in the evolution of these superficial variants, the abnormal melanocytes have not acquired the qualities that favor survival and progressive growth in the dermis. They are sensitive to immune processes that are operative in the papillary dermis. By repeated exposure to dermal immune processes, clones of resistant cells may be selected. The stages of radial spread (Level I and II) are expressions of evolving clones of melanocytes that have not acquired the properties that permit survival and propagation in the dermis. During this period of evolution, the papillary dermis may undergo significant thickening (reactive stroma).

Clones of neoplastic melanocytes that have acquired resistance and are capable of survival and propagation in the dermis aggregate in compact nests and fascicles to produce a local tumefaction. Survival in the dermis is not synonymous with active invasion of the reticular dermis. Some resistant clones may grow at the surface of the reticular dermis to produce a polypoid lesion that abuts on the reticular dermis. The interface between tumor and reticular dermis may be relatively straight or concave. Lesions of this type (polypoid Level III) may metastasize, but in general have a better prognosis than tumors that actively invade the reticular dermis. The acquisition of resistance by a clone of neoplastic melanocytes need not be a stepwise process. In some melanomas, resistance is an early or immediate property, which permits the formation of a tumor nodule without a phase of superficial lateral growth. This property of immediate resistance is characteristic of the nodular malignant melanoma. The polyclonism of melanomas is often a feature of the vertical growth phase of superficial spreading melanoma (Fig. 6-34).

Melanomas may grow in an expansile pushing fashion with compression of the reticular dermis (Fig. 6-20), or they may grow in an infiltrating fashion with disruption of collagen bundles of the reticular dermis (Figs. 6-21 and 6-35). The evaluation of the interface between a nodule of melanoma cells and the underlying reticular dermis may be difficult. Inflammatory infiltrates may obscure this interface. In addition, collagen bundles of the reticular dermis may be lysed in advance of an enlarging nodule of melanoma and replaced by an inflamed or fibrotic granulation tissue stroma. In the face of such a dilemma it may be helpful to relate the deep margin of the tumor to normal structures in the adjacent dermis. If the deep margin is at or below the level of sebaceous glands, the tumor probably has extended into the reticular dermis even though tumor cells cannot be demonstrated between collagen bundles of the reticular dermis.

In the evolution of the ordinary acquired cellular nevus, the nevus cells migrate from the epidermis into the papillary dermis, which hypertrophies in response to the migrating nevus cells to form their stroma. The ordinary

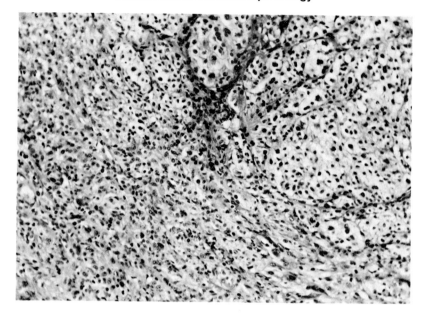

Fig. 6-34. Malignant melanoma showing regional variations in pattern (poly-clonism). On the left-hand side of the field the tumor cells have nevus cell charac-teristics and small slightly atypical nuclei. On the right-hand side of the field the tumor cells are arranged in nests and show a significant amount of nuclear atypism. The tumor cells within the nests have slightly vacuolated cytoplasm.

cellular nevus, in which the migration of nevus cells into the reticular dermis is limited is a lesion of the adventitial dermis. The polypoid mela-noma (Level III invasion) recapitulates the migration of nevus cells and the hypertrophy of the papillary dermis (adventitial dermis). The capacity to invade the reticular dermis is not peculiar to malignant melanocytes. This property is also characteristic of the proliferating melanocytes in a Spitz tumor (spindle cell nevus). The spindle cell nevus is distinguished by loosely arranged fascicles and by progressive maturation of tumor cells in the deep margin of the lesion. A spindle cell melanoma that has invaded the reticular dermis usually contains one or more nodules in which mela-nocytes are crowded together without regard for the stroma.

Breslow has presented evidence that the volume of the nodular portion of a malignant melanoma correlates with prognosis. At a practical level he has shown that a single measurement of the vertical size of the nodule offers prognostically and therapeutically significant information. Lesions whose vertical height is less than 0.76 mm are unlikely to metastasize. Breslow's observations offer additional evidence that the capacity of tumor

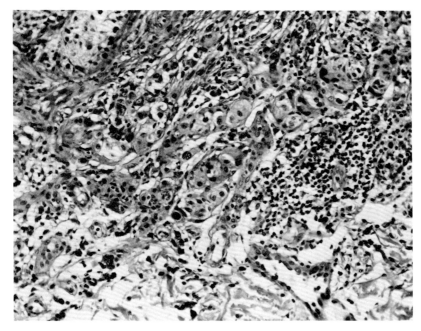

Fig. 6-35. Lower margin of a malignant melanoma showing extensions of fascicles of tumor cells between collagen bundles of the reticular dermis (Level IV invasion).

cells to survive in the dermis is related to the formation of a tumor nodule and in turn determines prognosis. In practice this measurement greatly aids in the evaluation of tumors at Level III invasion. There is recent evidence that lesions where height is greater than 1.5 mm are benefited by dissection of regional lymph nodes.

Borderline Melanocytic Lesions

The borderline melanocytic lesion is a common problem. These lesions are characterized by aggregates of cells that are loosely fasciculated in a delicate fibrous matrix. This matrix is indistinguishable from that of a benign nevus. The cells show minor degrees of nuclear atypism. Borderline tumors often show regional variation in pattern. Nests of slightly atypical nevus-like cells are commonly present at the deep margin of the tumor at the interface between tumor and reticular dermis. These cells are easily interpreted as remnants of a preexisting benign nevus but may be evidence of the polyclonism of melanomas. The tendency for malignant melanocytes to disregard their stroma and to aggregate in large nests is a feature of great value in evaluating borderline lesions. In addition, the nodules commonly show greater degrees of nuclear atypism (variation in nuclear size and staining, irregularities of nuclear membranes, nucleolar size, etc.) than adjacent nests of cells that are loosely arranged in fascicles that mimic the organoid pattern of a benign cellular nevus. The nodules are evidence of the polyclonism of melanomas and, in addition, are evidence that some of the clones have lost their nevus cell characteristics (fasciculation) and have acquired resistance.

PRIMARY LYMPHOHISTIOCYTIC RETICULOSIS OF THE SKIN

In most of the inflammatory processes that involve the skin, the inflammatory infiltrates are confined to the vascular adventitia, the papillary dermis, and the perifollicular connective tissue sheath. These anatomic divisions of the skin may be conveniently grouped as a functional unit, which is termed the adventitial dermis. In rare instances the adventitial dermis is involved by lymphohistiocytic disorders that are primary in the skin, are persistent, and may be locally progressive, evolve into a malignancy, or focally involute. An understanding of primary lymphohistiocytic reticuloses of the skin has been handicapped by clinical concepts that are archaic and controversial. Mycosis fungoides, parapsoriasis, and poikiloderma atrophicans vasculare are the three most common terms used to express clinically evolved concepts related to this group of disorders. At the histologic level these clinically evolved concepts are poorly defined. A useful histogenetic classification of these processes should give recognition to the following features:

1. Origin and distribution of infiltrates
2. Degree of lymphohistiocytic dysplasia
3. Natural history of infiltrates

By definition we are concerned with processes that are originally confined to the adventitial dermis. Under normal circumstances the adventitial dermis is sparsely cellular, but appears to represent a form of potential lymphoreticular tissue. In the primary lymphohistiocytic reticuloses the infiltrates appear to originate in the adventitial dermis by local proliferation of cells. The infiltrates usually appear first in the vascular adventitia and extend into other components of the adventitial dermis. They may become confluent and bandlike. They commonly extend to the epidermis and may be associated with focal degenerative changes in it.

In the classification of lymphohistiocytic reticuloses of the skin, recognition should be given to the degree of lymphohistiocytic dysplasia. Histologically and historically, the separation between parapsoriasis and mycosis fungoides is based in part on the absence of dysplasia in the former and its presence in the latter. In evaluating lymphohistiocytic dysplasia, emphasis is placed on the presence of atypical cells, their cytologic characteristics, and their numerical representation in proportion to cytologically benign components. The most significant cytologic component in these lymphohistiocytic dysplasias is a mononuclear cell with scanty cytoplasm and a convoluted, uniformly hyperchromatic nucleus (mycosis cell). This cell shows degrees of atypism that vary from a cell which is difficult to distinguish from a small histiocyte to a large cell with dense chromatin and a prominent nucleolus. It shares features at the ultrastructural level with Lutzner's cell, but its distinguishing feature of uniform nuclear hyperchromatism is not readily appreciated at the ultrastructural level. In some primary lymphohistiocytic dysplasias the mycosis cell is not a significant component of the infiltrate. In these disorders dysplasia is indicated by increasing immaturity of lymphohistiocytic cells comprising the infiltrate. In these examples the infiltrate contains a significant proportion of small reticulum cells. In some examples the nuclei of the small reticulum cells have plasmocytoid characteristics with prominent clumping of chromatin.

If atypical cells are not present in an infiltrate that satisfies the clinico-pathologic criteria for a primary lymphohistiocytic disorder, then it is qualified as lymphohistiocytic hyperplasia. The lymphohistiocytic dys-plasias may be graded as mild, moderate, or marked, depending on the cytologic characteristics and the proportion of atypical cells. If the infil-trate is composed entirely of ayptical cells (i.e., reticulum cells and mycosis cells or small reticulum cells) and is confined to the adventitial dermis, then it may be qualified as malignant reticulosis in situ. When the infil-trate breaks into the reticular dermis to form nodular aggregates or appears in extracutaneous sites such as lymph nodes, then it qualifies as malignant reticulosis-lymphohistiocytic variant (T-cell reticulosis?).

Parapsoriasis-Poikiloderma Complex

These lymphohistiocytic hyperplasias are characterized by bandlike infil-trates of lymphocytes and histiocytes in the adventitial dermis (Fig. 6-36). They are most characteristic when the infiltrates are confined to the papil-lary dermis. Occasionally the infiltrates are confined to the perifollicular connective tissue sheaths. They tend to hug the epidermis or the outer sheath of hair follicles. If they migrate into the epithelium, they are asso-ciated with degenerative changes in keratinocytes in the basal portions of these epithelial structures (lichenoid reaction). Rete ridges are often effaced (Fig. 6-37). Clefts are produced at the dermoepidermal interface

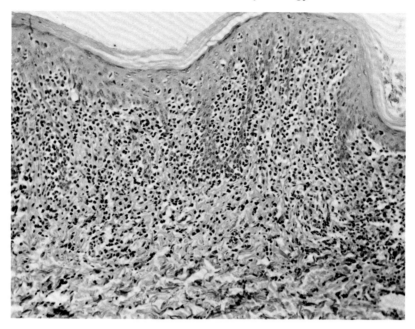

Fig. 6-36. Cellular phase of parapsoriasis-poikiloderma complex. Rete ridges are elongated but show attrition at the dermoepidermal interface with loss of the epidermal domain to the dermis (attrition-accretion phenomena). The infiltrate is lymphohistiocytic in character. The cells have somewhat irregular nuclear membranes and hyperchromatic nuclei. They tend to concentrate at the dermoepidermal junction, especially in sites showing evidence of attrition. Cells have also migrated into the stratum malpighii. The papillary dermis is slightly thickened.

(attrition of epidermis by dermal infiltrates). The clefts are subsequently incorporated into the dermis. This process is repeated in multiple sites and eventually results in thickening of the papillary dermis (accretive hyperplasia of papillary dermis). This type of lymphohistiocytic hyperplasia is additionally characterized by focal involution of the infiltrate. Where this has occurred, the adventitial dermis is thickened and contains an increased number of ectatic blood vessels (poikiloderma) (Fig. 6-38). In summary, the process is characterized by (1) lymphohistiocytic infiltrates (parapsoriasiform pattern), (2) attrition of epidermis and accretion of adventitial dermis (lichenoid reaction), and (3) focal involution of infiltrate (poikiloderma pattern). This histologic definition embraces most of the syndromes included under the heading of the parapsoriasis-poikiloderma complex.

Varying degrees of atypism may be present in the infiltrate of lesions

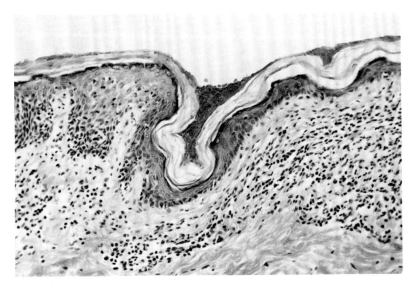

Fig. 6-37. Parapsoriasis-poikiloderma complex showing progression of the attrition-accretion phenomena. The fibrous expansion of the papillary dermis is at the expense of the epidermis. It is indicated in part by effacement of rete ridges. Prominent infiltrates are present in the thickened papillary dermis but are somewhat focal in distribution. There is no atypism in the infiltrates. This lesion shows changes that are intermediate between those of the cellular phase and the fibrotic phase of the parapsoriasis-poikiloderm complex.

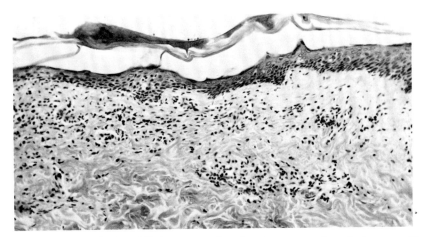

Fig. 6-38. Parapsoriasis-poikiloderma complex showing progression of changes with accentuation of papillary dermal fibrosis. The fibrous thickening of the papillary dermis is accompanied by a reduction in the lymphohistiocytic infiltrate and by evidence of attrition at the dermoepidermal junction (effacement of rete ridges).

in the parapsoriasis-poikiloderma complex (Fig. 6-39). The degree of dysplasia that should be indicated in the histologic diagnosis is measured by the proportion of atypical monocytoid cells.

Sezary Syndrome (Erythrodermic T-Cell Dysplasia)

In some examples of primary cutaneous lymphohistiocytic dysplasia there is relatively little evidence of focal involution. In these lesions the infiltrates diffusely fill a thickened papillary dermis (Figs. 6-40 and 6-41). They may distend the papillary dermis to a thickness four or more times greater than normal. This type of process may be associated with an erythroderma and with circulating atypical mononuclear cells in the blood (Sezary cells). The latter cells are similar to or identical with mycosis cells and, in combination with other features, define Sezary's syndrome (dermatopathic leukemia).

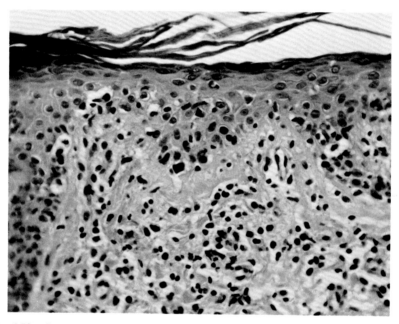

Fig. 6-39. Parapsoriasis-poikiloderma complex showing evidence of the attrition-accretion phenomena with partial effacement of rete ridges and fibrosis of the papillary dermis. The infiltrate is not dense but is characterized by the presence of atypical monocytoid cells in the epidermal portion. The epidermis has the features seen in lichenoid reactions. This represents an example of the parapsoriasis-poikiloderma complex with a mild degree of lymphohistiocytic dysplasia.

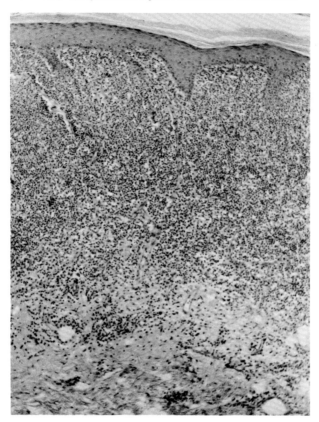

Fig. 6-40. Primary hyperplastic lymphohistiocytic reticulosis showing marked thickening of the papillary dermis with a dense bandlike infiltrate. The epedermis shows partial effacement of rete ridges but there is no significant infiltration of the epidermis by the lymphohistiocytic infiltrate. The infiltrate, which is lymphohistiocytic in character and shows little or no dysplasia, spills into the upper portion of the reticular dermis. Infiltrates of this type may be seen in the Sezary syndrome.

Psoriasiform Lymphohistiocytic Hyperplasia and Dysplasia

The second major group of primary lymphohistiocytic disorders is characterized by psoriasiform patterns in the epidermis (acanthosis and regular elongation of rete ridges) (Figs. 6-42 through 6-46). In this group varying degrees of lymphohistiocytic dysplasia are almost invariably present and the dysplastic cells are most evident in the epidermis. They usually infiltrate the epidermis as single cells, but may aggregate to form microabscesses (Pautrier microabscess) (Figs. 6-47 and 6-48). Similar cells are present in the dermis. They are mixed with nonspecific inflammatory cells

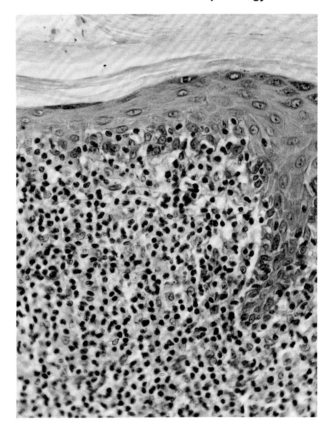

Fig. 6-41. A higher magnification of a primary lymphohistiocytic hyperplastic reticulosis shows the cytologically benign character of the infiltrate with relatively little invasion of the epidermis.

and may be difficult to identify. Varying reaction patterns may be seen in the papillary dermis in this group of disorders. The most common alteration is lamellar hyperplasia of fibrous tissue in the papillary dermis. This is a common reaction pattern that is most often seen in biopsies of lichen simplex chronicus. The psoriasiform pattern of primary lymphohistiocytic dysplasia is the histologic counterpart of the clinical syndrome known as mycosis fungoides.

In either the parapsoriasiform or the psoriasiform categories the infiltrate may be cytologically malignant (atypical and monomorphic), but confined to the adventitial dermis. As indicated earlier, this pattern is best

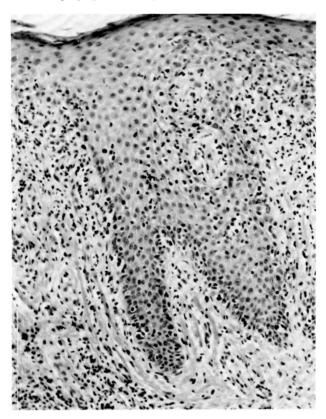

Fig. 6-42. Psoriasiform lymphohistiocytic dysplasias showing a psoriasiform pattern of epidermal hyperplasia and lamellar papillary dermal fibrosis. The infiltrate in the papillary dermis is rather loose and contains an occasional atypical monocytoid cell. The atypical monocytoid cells are more prominent in the epidermal infiltrate than in the dermal infiltrate. This represents a psoriasiform pattern with mild lymphohistiocytic dysplasia—a pattern most often seen in the clinical setting of the Alibert type of mycosis fungoides.

classified as malignant reticulosis in situ. Occasionally a biopsy of a lesion early in the clinical course of a lymphohistiocytic dysplasia shows the pattern of malignant reticulosis in situ. The implication from this finding is that the disorder has taken origin de novo as a cytologically malignant infiltrate. It is necessary to recognize this de novo, in situ variant (de novo reticulosis) and to distinguish it from examples of malignant reticulosis in situ that have evolved from a hyperplasia or dysplasia (evolved reticulosis).

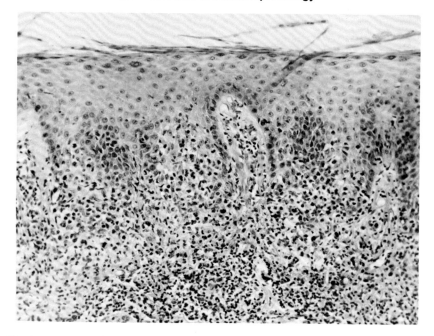

Fig. 6-43. Psoriasiform lymphohistiocytic dysplasia showing an overlap in features with lesions of the parapsoriasis-poikiloderma complex. There is evidence of attrition-accretion at the dermoepidermal interface. The degree of dysplasia is mild and is most evident in the epidermal portion of the infiltrate.

Malignant Cutaneous Reticulosis

Malignant cutaneous reticulosis refers to lymphohistiocytic disorders that are locally aggressive (invade the reticular dermis) or have spread to involve structures other than the skin, such as lymph nodes or viscera. Malignant cutaneous reticulosis may have evolved from a primary dysplasia or from a malignant reticulosis in situ. More often it is a manifestation of cutaneous involvement by a disseminated lymphoma of lymph nodal or visceral origin. Rarely a malignant cutaneous reticulosis arises de novo in the skin without evidence that it has either evolved from a local dysplasia, or from an in situ process, or has taken origin in a lymph node or in the viscera. If a grenz zone is present between the epidermis and the tumor, the process is probably a secondary cutaneous lymphoma. If the infiltrate extends to the epidermis, it may be evidence of a primary cutaneous malignant reticulosis (Fig. 6-49).

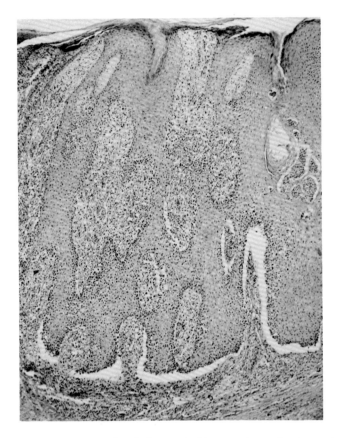

Fig. 6-44. An extreme example of the psoriasiform variant of primary lymphohistiocytic dysplasia. The infiltrate is pleomorphic and contains atypical monocytoid cells. These cells are more easily identified in the epidermal infiltrate than in the dermal infiltrate. The infiltrate is confined to a thickened papillary dermis and to the overlying epidermis.

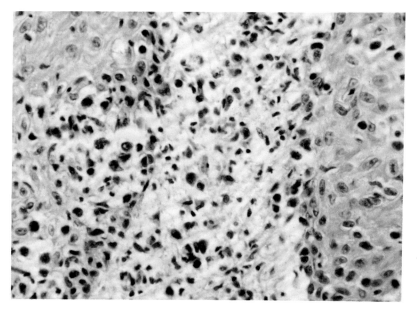

Fig. 6-45. High magnification of the lesion illustrated in Fig. 6-44. Atypical-mono-cytoid cells are present in the dermal infiltrate and in the epidermal infiltrate. In the epidermis some cells are clustered in poorly outlined microabscesses (Pautrier micro-abscesses).

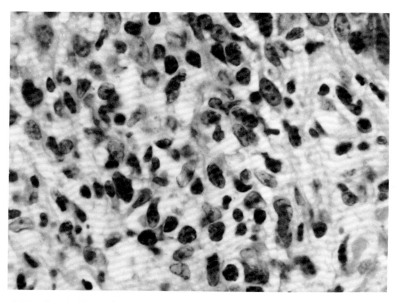

Fig. 6-46. Psoriasiform lymphohistiocytic dysplasia showing atypical monocytoid cells in the dermal infiltrate. The degree of dysplasia is slight to moderate.

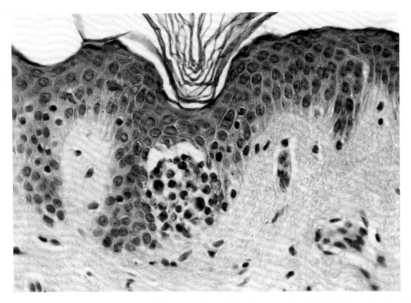

Fig. 6-47. A striking example of a Pautrier microabscess in which the typical cells are concentrated in loci in the epidermis with almost complete sparing of the papillary dermis.

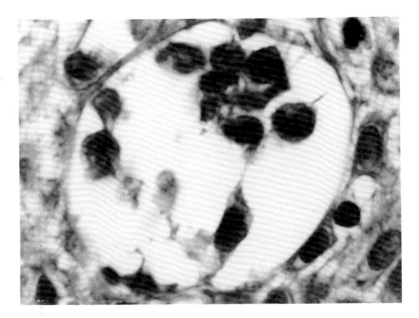

Fig. 6-48. Pautrier microabscess in a lesion of psoriasiform lymphohistiocytic dysplasia. The nuclei of the atypical monocytoid cells have folded convoluted nuclear membranes and are rather uniformly hyperchromatic. The atypical cells have a thin rim of cytoplasm.

107

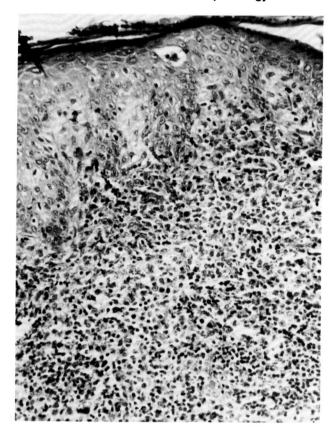

Fig. 6-49. Primary malignant cutaneous reticulosis showing a rather monotonous infiltrate of atypical mononuclear cells in a thickened papillary dermis. The infiltrate presses upon the epidermis and in some areas has migrated into it. The involvement of the epidermis by the abnormal dermal infiltrate is evidence favoring an interpretation that the process is primary in the skin rather than a manifestation of a systemic lymphoma.

Clinicopathologic Correlations

Patients whose lesions show the pattern of lymphohistiocytic hyperplasia usually present the clinical picture of either parapsoriasis or poikiloderma atrophicans vasculare. The clinical distinction between the latter two disorders is nebulous. If the histologic pattern is lichenoid with features of attrition-accretion, but also shows varying degrees of lymphohistiocytic dysplasia, the classification of the process according to classic concepts is complicated. The dysplastic component in the infiltrate may provide support for a histologic diagnosis of mycosis fungoides in a process that clinically is best classified as parapsoriasis-poikiloderma complex.

Not all of the disorders classified clinically as parapsoriasis qualify as primary lymphohistiocytic hyperplasias. This is particularly true of some of the processes classified as parapsoriasis en plaque. The latter term has been used for disorders showing nonspecific histologic patterns (perivascular infiltrates of chronic inflammatory cells) and for premalignant processes (parapsoriasis-poikiloderma complex). The examples that have nonspecific histologic changes are best classified as superficial chronic dermatitis. The term parapsoriasis should be reserved for primary lymphohistiocytic hyperplasia. The parapsoriasiform lesions (bandlike infiltrates) with lymphohistiocytic dysplasia may present clinically as an erythroderma. Atypical cells may be present in the blood (Sezary cells) and presumably have their origin in the dermal infiltrates (dermatopathic leukemia). The extremes of a clinical classification of parapsoriasis are well illustrated in Table 6-1 (Wise).

The psoriasiform lesions with lymphohistiocytic dysplasia generally correlate with clinical patterns recognized as the Alibert type of mycosis fungoides. This disease process is persistent and locally progressive. Characteristically lesions in this category evolve slowly, with progression from macules to plaques to tumors. In the tumor stage, the implication has been that the process has evolved into an outright malignancy (malignant reticulosis). In practice, a lesion that clinically is a tumor may show the histologic pattern of lymphohistiocytic dysplasia, malignant reticulosis in situ, or malignant reticulosis. If reliance is placed on clinical presentation, some of these patients will be treated aggressively at a period when the infiltrate does not qualify as a fully evolved malignancy.

Clinical Implications of Histologic Categories

It is implied in our classification of lymphohistiocytic hyperplasias and dysplasias (Table 6-2) that clinical progression of disease is accompanied by progressive dedifferentiation of the infiltrates. However, with the exception of occasional cases, it is difficult to document the histologic progression of lymphohistiocytic hyperplasias (Figs. 6-50 through 6-53). One of the major difficulties encountered in the study of this group of diseases is the iatrogenic termination of disease (and life) before it has run its natural course. As the pathologist with the examination of successive specimens becomes more secure in his diagnosis, the clinician becomes more vigorous in his efforts to eradicate the disease.

The lymphohistiocytic hyperplasias and dysplasias generally are chronic, relatively benign diseases. It is difficult or impossible to correlate the his-

Table 6-1

Parapsoriasis (Wise)
(Historical)

1890	Parakeratosis Variegata	Unna, Santi and Pollitzer
1894	Dermatitis Psoriasiformis Nodularis	Neisser
1894	Psoriasiform and Lichenoid Exanthem	Jadassohn
1897	Pityriasis Lichenoides Chronica	Juliusberg
1897	Erythrodermie Pityriasique en Plaques Disseminees	Brocq
1900	Lichen Variegatus	Crocker
1900	Brocq's Disease	Arndt
1901	Chronic Resistant Macular and Maculo-Papular Scaling Erythrodermias	Colcott Fox and MacLeod
1902	Scaling Erythrodermias Appearing in Disseminated Spots	Torok
1902	Parapsoriasis en goutes	Brocq
	Parapsoriasis lichenoide	Brocq
	Parapsoriasis en plaques	Brocq
1903	Parapsoriasis nodularis	Bucek
1903	Parapsoriasis maculosa	Bucek
1903	Parapsoriasis mixta	Bucek
1905	Xantho-Erythrodermia Perstans	Crocker and White, and Pernet
1906	Pityriasis Maculosa Chronica	Rusch
1907	Erythrodermia Maculosa Perstans (or Chronica)	Riecke
1924	Erythrodermie Polymorphe Persistante	Gastou
	Dermatitis variegata	Boeck
	Dermatosi squamosi anormale	Casoli
	Morbus Jadassohni	Rona
	Parapsoriasis Atrophicans	Kreibich
	Pityriasis Lichenoides et Varioliformis Acuta	Habermann

tologic patterns with the rate of progression of disease. Occasionally it is possible to document rapid progression from a dysplasia to an in situ reticulosis to a malignant reticulosis. In many cases the histologic pattern remains relatively stable over long periods of time. For those processes that are confined to the adventitial dermis, there is little or no likelihood of systemic spread of disease. Clinical management should be conservative and cautious. Vigorous therapy under the mistaken notion that the diagnosis of mycosis fungoides always implies a fully evolved malignant lymphoreticulosis may be disasterous for the patient.

Occasionally lymphohistiocytic hyperplasias may invade the reticular

Table 6-2
**Cutaneous Lymphoreticulosis
(including T-cell hyperplasias and dysplasias)**

Classification
  I. Primary cutaneous lymphohistiocytic (T-cell) hyperplasia and dysplasia (attrition-accretion variant; parapsoriasis-poikiloderma complex; mycosis fungoides, erythrodermic variant; Sezary syndrome)
     A. minimal or no dysplasia
     B. moderate dysplasia
     C. marked dysplasia
     D. dermatopathic leukemia (Sezary phenomenon) ±
 II. Primary cutaneous lymphohistiocytic (T-cell) hyperplasia and dysplasia (acanthotic-exocytotic variant; psoriasiform variant; mycosis fungoides-Alibert)
     A. minimal or no dysplasia
     B. moderate dysplasia
     C. marked dysplasia
     D. dermatopathic leukemia ±
III. Primary malignant reticulosis in situ (T-cell lymphoma) (confined to adventitial dermis)
     A. evolved (preceded by type I or II)
     B. de novo
     C. dermatopathic leukemia ±
 IV. Primary malignant reticulosis (T-cell lymphoma) (infiltration of reticular dermis; mycosis fungoides-d'emblée or evolved)
     A. evolved (preceded by type I, II, or III)
     B. de novo (d'emblée)
     C. dermatopathic leukemia ±
  V. Secondary malignant reticulosis (visceral or nodal lymphoma with cutaneous involvement)
 VI. Controversial and symptomatic lymphoreticuloses
     A. vascular reticuloses
         1. lymphomatoid papulosis
         2. lymphomatoid granulomatosis
         3. eosinophilic-histiocytic reticulosis
         4. eruptive phase, malignant cutaneous reticulosis
     B. follicular mucinosis
VII. Secondary lymphohistiocytic hyperplasias
     A. actinic reticuloid
     B. contact dermatitis
     C. viral diseases
VIII. Benign cutaneous lymphoplasia
     A. localized
     B. disseminated
 IX. Angioblastic lymphoid hyperplasia with eosinophilia
  X. Lymphocytic infiltrates of dermis
     A. erythema annulare centrifugum
     B. polymorphic light eruption
     C. lupus erythematosus
     D. drug eruption

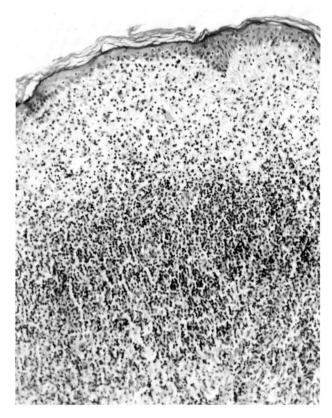

Fig. 6-50. Primary lymphohistiocytic hyperplastic reticulosis showing a markedly thickened papillary dermis containing a dense infiltrate of lymphocytes and small histiocytes. There is no evidence of lymphohistiocytic dysplasia.

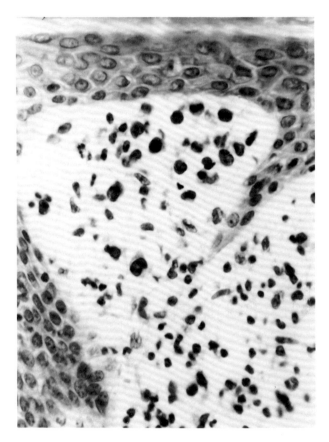

Fig. 6-51. Six years later in a lesion from the same patient as that illustrated in Fig. 6-50, the infiltrate is still confined to a thickened papillary dermis. It contains a moderate number of atypical monocytoid cells (moderate dysplasia).

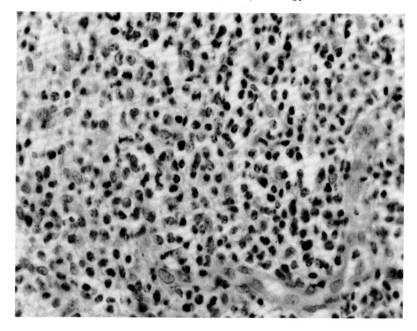

Fig. 6-52. Biopsy of a lesion in the same patient as that illustrated in Figs. 6-50 and 6-51. This biopsy was taken several months after the biopsy illustrated in Fig. 6-51. The infiltrate is composed of atypical histiocytes that show a plasmacytoid pattern of clumping of nuclear chromatin. Mitoses are present. There has been a reduction in the number of lymphocytes in the infiltrate, and this combination of progressive dysplasia and lymphocyte depletion might be compared to a similar process that occurs in Hodgkin's disease.

dermis but maintain a relatively benign cytologic character. The "tumor stage" of mycosis fungoides may not show a significant degree of dedifferentiation (Fig. 6-54). Cases of this type are too rare to make any general statements regarding their prognosis.

Lymphohistiocytic Hyperplasias (Lymph Node Patterns)

The lymph node reactions in primary lymphohistiocytic hyperplasias of the skin share cytologic features with the dermal infiltrates. They are generally classified as dermatopathic lymphadenitis (lipophagic melanotic reticulosis). The changes, which primarily involve the tissue between sinusoids and germinal centers, are characterized by diffuse infiltrates of pale histiocytes with a sprinkling of plasma cells and eosinophiles (Fig. 6-55). Bordering the aggregates of histiocytes, the medullary tissue is hyper-

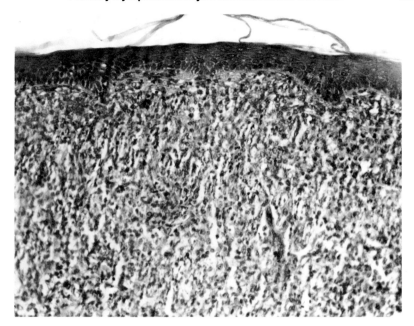

Fig. 6-53. Later sequential biopsy from same patient as the lesions illustrated in Figs. 6-50, 6-51, and 6-52. At this stage in the evolution of the disease there has been almost complete lymphocyte depletion. The infiltrate, which is composed of small atypical histiocytes, is separated from the epidermis by a band of uninvolved connective tissue. At this stage the distinction between primary and secondary cutaneous reticulosis is lost.

plastic and contains a variable number of lymphoblasts (Fig. 6-56). Mitoses may be present in the histiocytic component or in the hyperplastic lymphoid tissue.

In a general way these nodal histiocytic infiltrates mirror the cytologic characteristics of the dermal infiltrates. With progressive dysplasia in the dermal lymphohistiocytic infiltrates, there may be a corresponding dysplasia involving the lymphohistiocytic infiltrates in the lymph nodes. This lymph node reaction is an additional manifestation of the lymphohistiocytic dysplasia that is primarily evident in the skin.

Histogenetic Implications

There are histologic similarities between inflammatory processes of the lichenoid type and primary lymphohistiocytic hyperplasias, particularly those in the parapsoriasis-poikiloderma complex. The histologic pattern

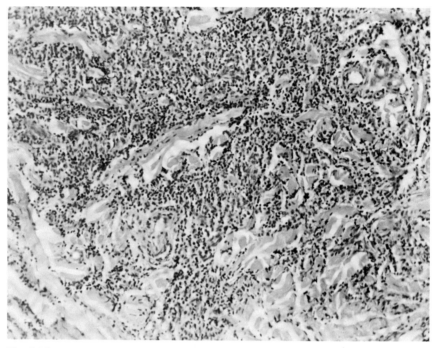

Fig. 6-54. Primary cutaneous reticulosis showing an infiltrate of small lymphocytes and histiocytes in the reticular dermis. The infiltrate extends between collagen bundles of the reticular dermis. There is little or no evidence of a lymphohistiocytic dysplasia. At the margins of this area of reticular dermal infiltration, the infiltrate was bandlike and limited to the papillary dermis, where it had the characteristics of a primary cutaneous lymphohistiocytic hyperplasia. The infiltrate has acquired the capacity to invade the reticular dermis but the invasive properties are not accompanied by a significant lymphohistiocytic dysplasia or by lymphocyte depletion. Lesions of this type are rare and for some reason appear to be more commonly localized to the lower extremities.

seen in lichen planus is the archtype of lichenoid reactions. It is characterized by degeneration and attrition of keratinocytes and accretion of papillary dermal connective tissue at the dermoepidermal interface. Colloid bodies that are effete keratinocytes are markers of the attrition-accretion interplay. Similar lichenoid patterns may be seen in lichenoid keratoses (inflamed actinic and seborrheic keratoses) and in some drug eruptions (atabrine reactions). Some processes that are clinically categorized as examples of lichen planus are chronic and persistent and show areas of poikiloderma. It is difficult to make a clear separation between lichen planus-like lesions of the latter type and primary lymphohistiocytic hyperplasias of the parapsoriasis-poikiloderma complex.

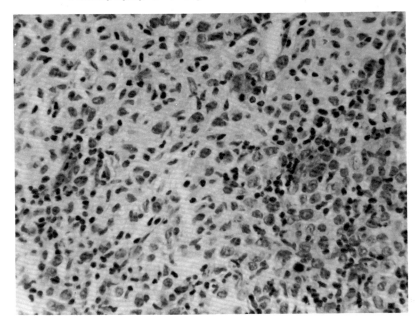

Fig. 6-55. Dermatopathic lymphadenitis in a patient with a psoriasiform pattern of lymphohistiocytic dysplasia (moderate dysplasia). The reaction in the lymph node is characterized by aggregates of pale histiocytes with an abundant amount of cytoplasm. Occasional atypical monocytoid cells are present in the infiltrate. Bordering the aggregates of histiocytes, the lymph node shows immature cells of the lymphoid series. The nodal infiltrates tend to mirror those in the skin but may not show the same degree of dysplasia.

It is generally assumed that the defect in lymphohistiocytic hyperplasias (parapsoriasis-poikiloderma complex) resides in the lymphoreticular tissues. From the evidence derived from a histologic study of epidermal changes and of the distribution of infiltrates in lichenoid reactions and in lymphohistiocytic hyperplasias, it could be argued that the primary defect may reside in the epidermis. The basal layer of the epidermis (basal keratinocytic-melanocytic system) appears to suffer the greatest damage in the attrition-accretion reaction (Fig. 6-57).

In many examples of lymphohistiocytic dysplasias, the mycosis cells often are most numerous and most easily identified in the epidermal infiltrates (Figs. 6-58 and 6-59). They lose their identity and are relatively obscured by other inflammatory cells in the dermal infiltrates. Either the mycosis cells are reacting to "defective" keratinocytes or they are relatively protected in the epidermis from immune processes of the host. The pleomorphism of the infiltrates in the dermis has been interpreted as an

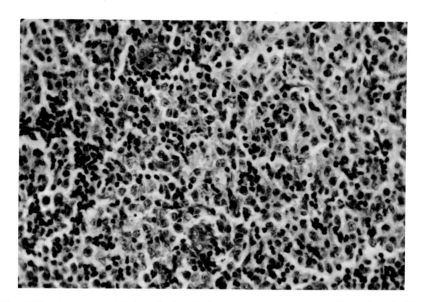

Fig. 6-56. Dermatopathic lymphadenitis in a patient with psoriasiform lymphohistiocytic dysplasia. Immature lymphocytes are present in the lymph node bordering aggregates of pale histiocytes.

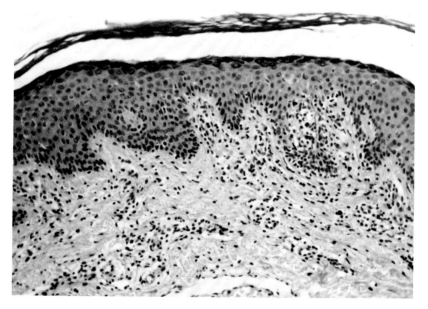

Fig. 6-57. Parapsoriasis-poikiloderma complex showing a significant amount of papillary dermal fibrosis with mild perivascular infiltrates of lymphocytes and histiocytes. The infiltrate tends to aggregate at the dermoepidermal interface, where it is associated with degenerative changes in basal keratinocytes.

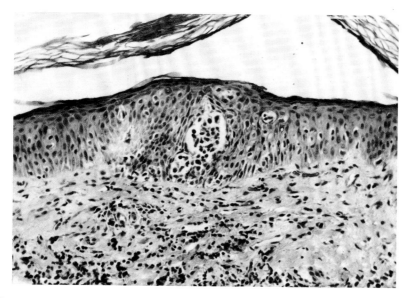

Fig. 6-58. Lymphohistiocytic dysplasia showing rather striking aggregates of atypical monocytoid cells in the epidermis. Similar cells are difficult to identify in the dermal infiltrates. This is often a feature of infiltrates in lesions of the parapsoriasis-poikiloderma complex and in lesions of the psoriasiform variant of lymphohistiocytic hyperplasia and dysplasia. This lesion is difficult to categorize as either the parapsoriasis-poikiloderma complex or the psoriasiform variant.

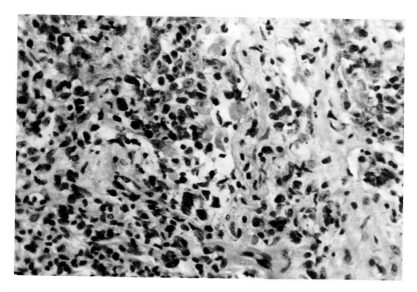

Fig. 6-59. Lymphohistiocytic dysplasia showing a moderate degree of dysplasia. The dysplastic atypical monocytoid cells are more easily identified in the epidermal infiltrates than in the dermis.

119

expression of an immune process directed against an abnormal clone of lymphoreticular cells.

It is sometimes difficult to make a sharp distinction between primary lymphohistiocytic hyperplasias (Fig. 6-60) and reactive hyperplasias, such as lichen simplex chronicus (Fig. 6-61).

Vascular Reticuloses

We have defined a group of lymphohistiocytic hyperplasias and dysplasias that are characterized by a predilection for the adventitial dermis, particularly the papillary and perifollicular dermis. There remains a heterogene-

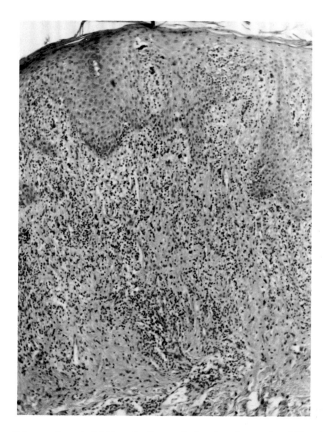

Fig. 6-60. Primary lymphohistiocytic hyperplasia showing a bandlike infiltrate of lymphocytes and histiocytes in a thickened fibrotic papillary dermis. The infiltrate shows no degree of dysplasia. Lesions of this type may be difficult to distinguish from lichen simplex chronicus, contact dermatitis, or reactions to heavy metals.

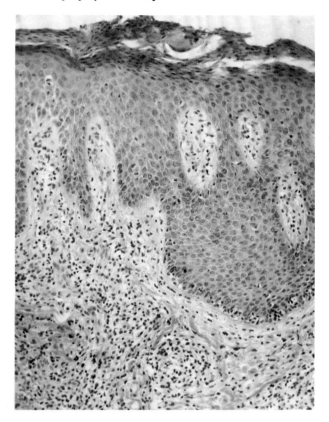

Fig. 6-61. Lymphohistiocytic hyperplasia not readily classifiable as a primary cutaneous reticulosis. There is a significant degree of papillary dermal fibrosis and a thickening of the papillary dermis. Patterns of this type may be seen in severe contact dermatitis and in lichen simplex chronicus. A similar pattern may sometimes be seen in inflamed tatoos.

ous group in which atypical infiltrates are more or less confined to dermal vascular adventitia and are often associated with degeneration, inflammation, and necrosis of the involved vessels. The term vascular reticulosis has been selected as a generic name for this heterogeneous group. Included in this group are recurrent self-limited processes that are classified as lymphomatoid papulosis. The infiltrates of follicular mucinosis, some lesions of cutaneous Hodgkin's disease, eruptive phases of cutaneous malignant reticulosis (Fig. 6-62), and some less well-defined disorders are included in this group. The cutaneous lesions of lymphomatoid granulomatosis might also be characterized as a vascular reticulosis. Not all of these

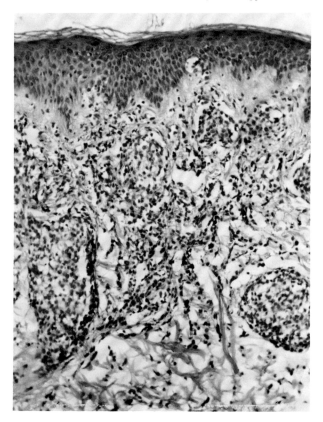

Fig. 6-62. Eruptive phase in the evolution of primary cutaneous malignant reticulosis. Biopsies of lesions early in the evolution of the disease showed a pattern compatible with a primary malignant reticulosis of the skin. Late in the evolution of the disease, the patient presented an eruption of macules and papules. This section is representative of a biopsy of one of the eruptive lesions. The infiltrate, which is almost entirely perivascular and more or less confined to the reticular dermis, is composed of small atypical histiocytes.

processes are self-limited. Some, such as cutaneous Hodgkin's disease, may be locally destructive, showing necrosis and sloughing of involved tissue.

Lymphomatoid Papulosis

The problem of the vascular reticuloses is exemplified by the syndrome of lymphomatoid papulosis. This process originally was characterized as a variant of pityriasis lichenoides et varioliformis acuta (PLVA). This is a good example of the troublesome terminology facing the trainee in dermatopathology. Such terminology is descriptive of clinical characteristics, but offers little or no insight into histogenesis. Included within this clinical syndrome were rare processes that histologically share features with ordinary forms of PLVA, but cytologically are distinctive. For this group of cytologically atypical processes the term lymphomatoid papulosis is currently popular. Epidermal infiltrates are a consistent feature of PLVA, but are a variable feature of lymphomatoid papulosis. Perivascular infiltrates are characteristic of both disorders.

The infiltrate in lymphomatoid papulosis is cytologically atypical and pleomorphic. In some examples the infiltrates are cytologically malignant. Many of the cells have the features of mycosis cells. Bizarre reticulum cells with large hyperchromatic irregular nuclei are present in the perivascular infiltrates, in the interstitial spaces of the reticular dermis, in the papillary dermis, and in the epidermis. If epidermal involvement is a significant feature, the reaction takes on some or many of the characteristics of mycosis fungoides. The vessels in a lesion of lymphomatoid papulosis usually are involved and may show focal areas of fibrinoid necrosis. Lymphomatoid papulosis is distinguished by the rapid evolution of individual lesions. Over a period of weeks or months the lesions involute and terminate in complete resolution.

In occasional lesions, the infiltrate is monomorphic, diffuse, and composed of primitive stem cells or small reticulum cells (Figs. 6-63, 6-64 and 6-65). Cytologically lesions of this type are malignant lymphomas. These lesions may represent an eruptive stage of a malignant reticulosis. They are distinguished by their perivascular distribution and by relatively rapid spontaneous resolution.

It is implied in the concept and nosology of lymphomatoid papulosis that the process is chronic, but benign and self-limited. Cases with long term follow-up would tend to support this concept. A few examples have evolved into persistent cutaneous neoplasms that are indistinguishable from the evolved malignant lymphohistiocytic reticuloses. Lymphomatoid papulosis may be another example of lymphohistiocytic dysplasia that in occasional cases may evolve into a malignant reticulosis.

Lymphomatoid Granulomatosis

Lymphomatoid granulomatosis is a form of vascular reticulosis characterized by atypical lymphohistiocytic infiltrates that produce or are associated with necrosis of involved blood vessels. In many examples the infiltrates are cytologically malignant, but only occasional examples have progressed to a systemic malignant lymphoma. Although lesions of lymphomatoid

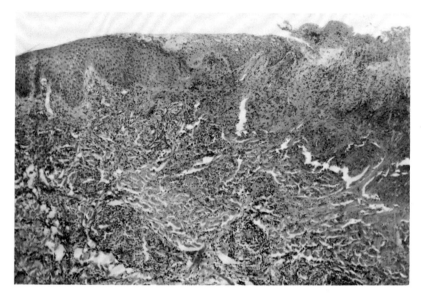

Fig. 6-63. Vascular reticulosis in a patient presenting the clinical pattern of lymphomatoid papulosis. A wedge-shaped area of infarction is present on the right-hand side of the field. Vessels in the adjacent viable dermis have thickened walls and are cuffed by infiltrates of atypical mononuclear cells that have histiocytic qualities.

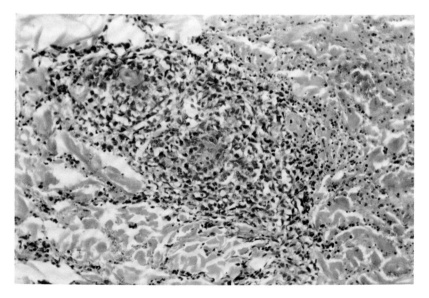

Fig. 6-64. Vascular reticulosis showing an infiltrate of atypical histiocytic cells in the perivascular spaces. The adjacent dermis is partially necrotic and contains nuclear debris. (Same lesion as Fig. 6-63.)

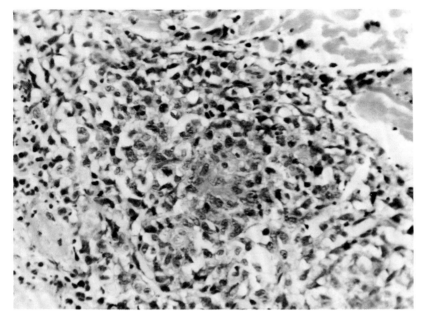

Fig. 6-65. High magnification showing the character of the infiltrating cells. The vessel has been partially occluded by the infiltrate and there is a small area of fibrinoid necrosis.

granulomatosis may be widespread, involvement of the lung is a requisite for the diagnosis. Approximately 50% of the patients with lymphomatoid granulomatosis will manifest skin lesions, some of which may call attention to silent pulmonary lesions. The lesions of lymphomatoid granulomatosis share features with those of midline reticulosis. The cutaneous lesions bear no resemblance to those of lymphomatoid papulosis. In the skin the infiltrates of lymphomatoid granulomatosis (Figs. 6-66 and 6-67) are perivascular. They are vasocentric and may be vasodestructive. They may infiltrate the blood vessels to produce partial or complete occlusion of the lumens. They tend to be prominent in the deeper portion of the dermis and extend into the subcutis. The involvement of the superficial portion of the dermis, which is often a characteristic feature of lymphomatoid papulosis, is apparently not a common feature of lymphomatoid granulomatosis. An angiitis with an infiltrate of benign inflammatory cells may occasionally be a feature of a malignant reticulosis (Fig. 6-68).

Eosinophilic-Histiocytic Reticulosis

A group of cutaneous disorders is characterized by perivascular infiltrates that are composed almost entirely of histiocytes with an admixture of

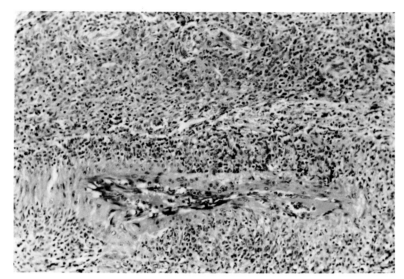

Fig. 6-66. Vascular reticulosis in a patient presenting the clinical picture of lymphomatoid granulomatosis. The infiltrate is vasocentric and vasodestructive. It is pleomorphic and contains atypical monocytoid cells, stem cells, and histiocytes. The vasodestructive quality is reflected in areas of infarction that are not illustrated in this field.

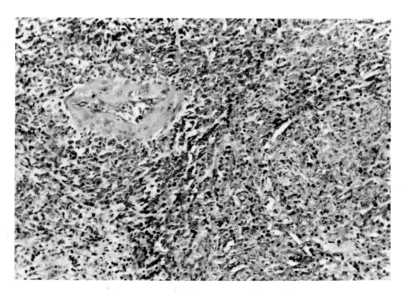

Fig. 6-67. Vascular reticulosis (same patient as Fig. 6-66) showing a monomorphic infiltrate of stem cells and atypical histiocytes. The infiltrate is vasocentric.

126

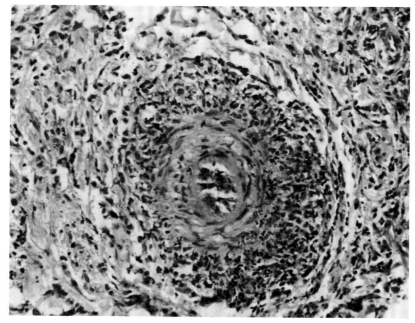

Fig. 6-68. Necrotizing vasculitis in a patient presenting a variety of cutaneous and oral mucosal lesions. Biopsies of a necrotic lesion on the dorsum of the tongue were interpreted as a pleomorphic reticulum cell sarcoma. The infiltrate was of a type that has been reported in midline reticulosis. Cutaneous lesions were characterized by a necrotizing vasculitis with granulomatous infiltrates outlining zones of necrosis. The histologic spectrum varied from that of midline reticulosis to Wegener's granulomatosis.

eosinophils. Lesions showing this histology may be localized and clinically may mimic mycosis fungoides. A similar histologic picture may be found in association with an erythroderma and clinically is associated with intense pruritus. These infiltrates may spill into the reticular dermis, but are most prominent in the perivascular spaces (Fig. 6-69). They may be associated with necrosis of the involved vessels. The infiltrates that are most prominent in the reticular dermis and the subcutis may be relatively inconspicuous in the papillary and perifollicular connective tissue sheaths. The histiocytic component shows varying degrees of atypism, but in many instances, the cells are cytologically benign. In those examples in which the infiltrate takes on atypical characteristics, the differential diagnosis includes cutaneous Hodgkin's disease (Fig. 6-70). This category of disorders shares some features with lymphomatoid granulomatosis and with allergic granulomatosis. Areas of necrotizing eosinophilic collagenosis may be a feature of the process in the dermis. A striking elevation of eosinophils

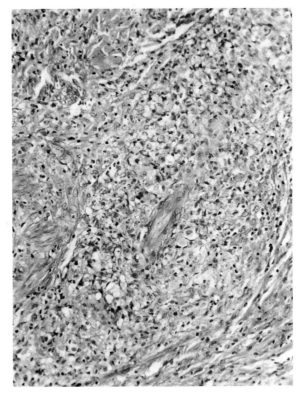

Fig. 6-69. Vascular reticulosis showing the histologic pattern of eosinophilic histiocytic reticulosis. The infiltrate is composed almost entirely of pale histiocytes with vacuolated cytoplasm and delicate nuclear membranes. Scattered eosinophils are present in the infiltrate and in the adjacent reticular dermis.

in the peripheral blood is often a prominent feature. The process is relatively rare and is too poorly defined to deserve additional comment.

SECONDARY LYMPHOHISTIOCYTIC HYPERPLASIAS

We have been primarily concerned with primary lymphohistiocytic hyperplasias of the skin. Over the years there has been a question whether banal inflammatory disorders such as psoriasis or pityriasis lichenoides et varioliformis acuta might occasionally evolve into a lymphohistiocytic dysplasia or neoplasia. If a lymphohistiocytic dysplasia or neoplasia takes origin in a preexisting inflammatory process, then it would qualify as an example of an intralesional transformation. It is extremely difficult to

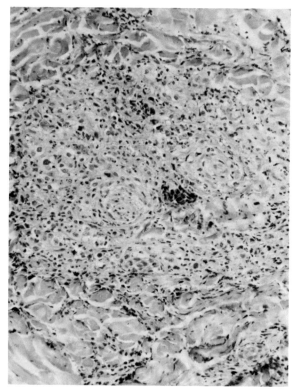

Fig. 6-70. Vascular reticulosis showing histologic features resembling those seen in eosinophilic histiocytic reticulosis. The patient was under treatment for advanced Hodgkin's disease and developed a cutaneous ulcer that destroyed a large part of the anterior chest wall. This biopsy is from the edge of such an ulceration. Some of the cutaneous lesions of Hodgkin's disease present the histologic pattern of the eosinophilic-histiocytic reticulosis.

document a transformation of the infiltrate of an inflammatory process to a dysplasia or a neoplasia. There is some evidence that this may occasionally occur in psoriasis, but in all likelihood these examples represent the psoriasiform type of primary lymphohistiocytic reticulosis in which the atypical changes are not well developed. There are processes characterized by dense lymphohistiocytic hyperplasias that may occasionally be confused with those of lymphohistiocytic dysplasias or neoplasias.

Actinic Reticuloid

A rare process described under the term of *actinic reticuloid* qualifies as an example of a lymphohistiocytic reaction that may mimic a reticulosis.

The lesions tend to be confined to areas exposed to the sun. They are characterized by dense lymphohistiocytic infiltrates showing varying degrees of immaturity in the reacting cells. These immature cells may be difficult to distinguish from those seen in lymphohistiocytic reticulosis. In general the lesions are characterized by psoriasiform patterns, but are distinguished from psoriasiform lymphohistiocytic dysplasias by an absence of significant atypism in the epidermal component of the infiltrate. In addition the epidermis often shows a degree of exudative changes seldom seen in primary lymphohistiocytic reticulosis. In actinic reticuloid the papillary dermis, which characteristically is thickened, shows rather striking degrees of lamellar hyperplasia. Multinucleated cells are often a prominent feature of the inflammatory infiltrate in the thickened papillary dermis.

Contact Dermatitis

Lymphohistiocytic hyperplasias of a degree which approaches that seen in actinic reticuloid may occasionally be seen in some examples of contact dermatitis. These processes may be difficult to distinguish from primary lymphohistiocytic dysplasias and neoplasias.

Viral Diseases

Viral diseases may occasionally be characterized by dense lymphohistiocytic infiltrates in the dermis, which often show varying degrees of immaturity. In some examples, such as herpetic infections, the reacting cells tend to be most prominent in the perivascular spaces and may be associated with necrosis of the involved vessels. If close attention is not paid to the necrotizing changes in the epidermis, this combination of features may suggest the possibility of a vascular reticulosis. Rather striking forms of lymphohistiocytic hyperplasia are seen in orf and milker's nodule (Figs. 6-71 and 6-72). The infiltrates, which may fill the upper portion of the dermis, show varying degrees of immaturity. The nuclear membranes of the immature cells are regular and do not show the striking convolutions seen in lymphohistiocytic dysplasias. Plasma cells are often a feature of this type of reactive lymphohistiocytic hyperplasia. The diagnosis is made by careful observation of the epidermis. In these disorders the epidermis generally is markedly hyperplastic and may show pseudoepitheliomatous hyperplasia. The inflammatory cells may migrate into the epidermis, but again they do not show the nuclear characteristics of a mycosis cell. In one or more areas the epidermal cells show degenerative changes. It is usually possible to find one or more areas either in the epidermis or in

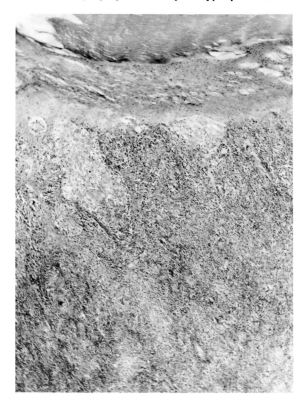

Fig. 6-71. Viral induced cutaneous lymphohistiocytic hyperplasia (milker's nodule). The epidermis shows parakeratosis, acanthosis, elongation of rete ridges, and intracellular and intercellular edema. The papillary dermis is markedly thickened and contains a dense bandlike infiltrate of inflammatory cells. The infiltrate is pleomorphic and is composed of lymphocytes, histiocytes, plasma cells, and primitive lymphoid cells. The primitive lymphoid cells may be prominent in lesions of this type and may be the source of confusion with atypical monocytoid cells of primary lymphohistiocytic dysplasias.

involved follicles in which the altered keratinocytes contain homogeneous acidophilic inclusions.

Follicular Mucinosis

Follicular mucinosis is a disease of pilosebaceous glands that is characterized by dedifferentiation of sebaceous glands and by the accumulation of a mucinous matrix in the interstices of follicular cells. The mucinous material may form pools in the outer sheath of the hair follicles. The primary

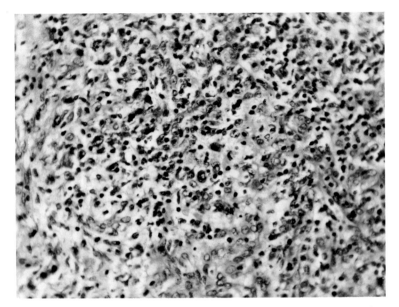

Fig. 6-72. Milker's nodule showing pleomorphic dermal infiltrate in which immature lymphoid cells are present.

form of the disease occurs as localized plaques or as disseminated widespread papular lesions. The adjacent dermis may be relatively free of
inflammatory infiltrates. In some lesions, prominent infiltrates of histiocytes, eosinophils, and reticulum cells are present in the adjacent dermis.
Histiocytes and eosinophiles may migrate into the areas of mucinous metaplasia in the involved follicles. These pleomorphic infiltrates are dense and
may be confused with those of a malignant reticulosis.

Follicular mucinosis may occur in lesions of primary cutaneous lymphohistiocytic dysplasia and malignant reticulosis. The association between
lymphohistiocytic dysplasias and symptomatic follicular mucinosis compli-
cates the interpretation of lesions of the primary form of follicular mucinosis that have dense pleomorphic perifollicular infiltrates. If the infiltrate
is not clearly a primary lymphohistiocytic dysplasia, a lesion of follicular
mucinosis is best considered to be a primary form of the disease rather
than a symptomatic variant.

BENIGN CUTANEOUS LYMPHOPLASIA

There are nodular lymphohistiocytic hyperplasias that involve the reticular
dermis and tend to spare the adventitial dermis. In this category are

lymphohistiocytic hyperplasias that are classified as benign cutaneous
lymphoplasia (benign lymphocytoma). The infiltrates in benign cutaneous lymphoplasia are pleomorphic. They are composed of lymphocytes,
histiocytes, reticulum cells, and a variable admixture of eosinophiles and
plasma cells (Fig. 6-73). They are usually most prominent in the deeper
portions of the reticular dermis and rarely involve the papillary dermis or
epidermis. Involvement of perifollicular sheaths and hair follicles is not a
prominent feature but occurs more commonly than involvement of the
epidermis. The histiocytes, which may be aggregated in irregular clusters,
occasionally form follicular aggregates that are indistinguishable from the
reaction centers of lymph nodes. The infiltrates extend along vessels into
the subcutaneous fat. Infiltration of the walls of venules at the deep margin

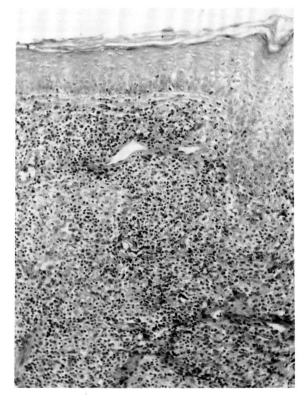

Fig. 6-73. Benign cutaneous lymphoplasia showing a pleomorphic dermal infiltrate
that is separated from the epidermis by a grenz zone. The infiltrate is composed of
lymphocytes and histiocytes. In some areas the histiocytes aggregate to produce a pattern resembling that seen in reaction centers. Some of the aggregated histiocytes may
have epithelioid qualities. This type of infiltrate may involve the walls of small veins
at the deep margin of the lesion.

of the dermis is a common feature. Hyaline deposits are often present in the dermal infiltrates. Vessels in the dermis in areas of infiltration are increased in number and have thickened walls and swollen endothelium. The distribution of the infiltrates and the absence of significant degrees of cytologic atypism distinguish benign cutaneous lymphoplasia from primary cutaneous malignant reticulosis. The pleomorphism of the infiltrate and the absence of cytologic atypism distinguish benign cutaneous lymphoplasia from secondary cutaneous reticulosis (Fig. 6-74). Disseminated forms of cutaneous lymphoplasia should be viewed with suspicion. Some of these will prove to be an early manifestation of a malignant lymphoma.

DIFFERENTIAL DIAGNOSIS (LYMPHOID LESIONS)

Perivascular Reactive Lymphocytic Infiltrates

The perivascular reactive lymphocytic infiltrates of the dermis may be difficult to distinguish from neoplastic infiltrates of lymphocytic leukemia.

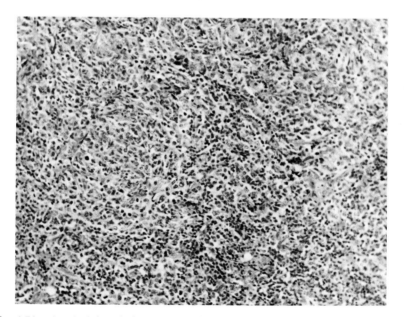

Fig. 6-74. Atypical lymphohistiocytic infiltrate in a cutaneous lesion on the temple of an elderly patient. The histiocytes, which are atypical, are aggregated in nodules and do not show phagocytosis of nuclear debris. Mitoses are present in the histiocytes. The nodules are separated from each other by a lymphoid stroma. Histologically the lesion qualifies as nodular lymphohistiocytic lymphoma. Lesions of this type are difficult to distinguish from benign cutaneous lymphoplasia.

The reactive infiltrates that are problems in differential diagnosis are characterized by a fairly uniform perivenular distribution in the reticular dermis. These infiltrates seldom have a significant component in the papillary dermis and usually spare the epidermis. Spotty infiltrates may occasionally extend into the epidermis. These processes are additionally distinguished by changes in the connective tissue of the reticular dermis. The collagen bundles may be fibrillated and are associated with an increased amount of mucinous matrix. In the areas in which collagenous alterations are prominent, the fibrocytes are hypertrophied and hyperplastic. In some forms (polymorphic light eruption, lymphocytic infiltrate of Jessner) the dermal connective tissue may be converted to a mucinous matrix. In some examples (polymorphic light eruption) the papillary dermis may be markedly edematous. Lupus erythematosus may occasionally be characterized by lymphocytic infiltrates in the reticular dermis. Usually the lesions in lupus erythematosus show significant and characteristic epidermal changes.

Secondary Lues

Secondary lues should be considered in the differential diagnosis of lymphohistiocytic hyperplasia. A diffuse bandlike infiltrate of lymphocytes and histiocytes in the papillary dermis that is accompanied by significant epidermal changes and by dense perivascular infiltrates in the dermis is characteristic of the reaction in secondary lues. Plasma cells are a variable component in the infiltrates.

Angioblastic Lymphoid Hyperplasia with Eosinophilia

Angioblastic lymphoid hyperplasia with eosinophilia is a rare lesion of unknown etiology. Lesions may be confined to the skin (atypical pyogenic granuloma); they may be multiple or solitary circumscribed subcutaneous tumors; or they may be multiple ill-defined subcutaneous tumors. In the dermis the lesions are circumscribed but not encapsulated. They are composed of tortuous vessels with thick laminated walls and swollen endothelium. The endothelial cells show variable degrees of nuclear atypism and many contain single distinct cytoplasmic vacuoles. The vessels are surrounded by an edematous fibrous matrix with scattered lymphoid aggregates. Eosinophiles are present in the lymphoid aggregates and in the fibrous matrix. The reaction in the papillary dermis and the epidermis is often indistinguishable from that seen in lichen simplex chronicus (psoriasiform epidermal hyperplasia and lamellar fibrosis of papillary dermis).

In the circumscribed subcutaneous lesion, the basic histologic features are the same as in those that are confined to the dermis, but are distinguished by a peculiar zonal variation in pattern (Fig. 6-75). The central

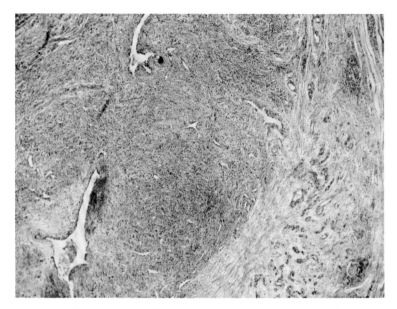

Fig. 6-75. Angioblastic lymphoid hyperplasia with eosinophilia showing zonal variation in pattern. There are two large angulated vascular spaces to the left of the center of the field. These spaces are surrounded by a circumscribed area containing numerous newly formed vessels and an infiltrate of lymphocytes. An aggregate of relatively mature loosely aggregated vessels is separated from the circumscribed nodule by a condensation of fibromuscular tissue. This condensation of tissue is interpreted as remnants of a preexisting vessel wall (probably artery) and apparently represents an aneurysmal dilatation of a preexisting vessel with marked angiogenesis in the aneurysmally dilated lumen and with extension of the newly formed vessels into adjacent soft tissue. In the adjacent soft tissue there is evidence of maturation. Lymphoid nodules, some of which contain reaction centers, are also present at the periphery of the lesion.

portion of such a lesion shows poorly formed vessels and a striking proliferation of plump atypical endothelial cells. It is often possible to identify a partially destroyed artery in or near the active center of the lesion (Fig. 6-76). Atypical proliferating endothelial cells may be traced from the lumen of this vessel, through its wall, into the vessels forming the lesion (Fig. 6-77). The periphery of such a lesion contains nodular lymphoid infiltrates and a plexus of relatively mature vessels. An intermediate zone may be distinguished in which there is progressive transformation of the newly formed vessels from the angioblastic swollen endothelial tubules in the central portion to the small thick-walled vessels at the periphery. Eosinophiles are present throughout the lesion.

In the disseminated variants, the lesions have ill-defined margins and

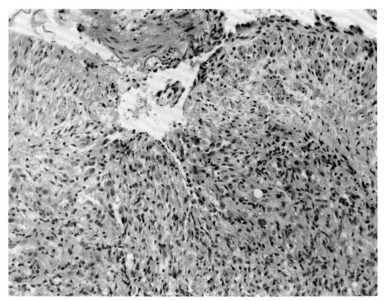

Fig. 6-76. A remnant of a muscular artery is present at the top of the field. Fragments of the wavy internal elastic lamina remain attached to the muscularis of the vessel, which is interrupted just above the center of the field. Tubules lined by plump atypical endothelial cells extend from the space separating the muscularis of the vessel into the adjacent tissue. Many of the cells have cytoplasmic vacuoles.

may infiltrate skeletal muscle. The lymphoid infiltrates in these lesions may be mistaken for those of a lymphoma.

IMMUNOLOGIC SUBCLASSES OF LYMPHOCYTES AND CUTANEOUS LYMPHOID INFILTRATES

The currently recognized immunologic subclasses of lymphocytes are B and T lymphocytes. This terminology compares each subclass to avian bursal and mammalian thymic lymphocytes. The mammalian equivalent of the avian bursal lymphocyte is typified by lymphoid tissue of Peyer's patches. Rather sophisticated studies are required to fully characterize a lymphoid reaction as involving one or both of these subclasses. The results of animal experiments and studies on lymphomas and immunodeficient diseases may be summarized as follows for each subgroup.

T lymphocytes
1. 70% of peripheral blood lymphocytes

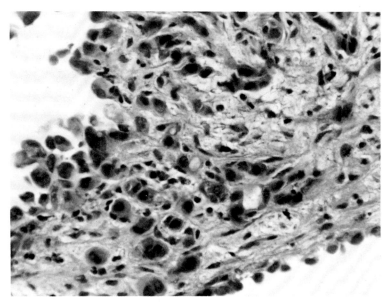

Fig. 6-77. The atypical character of the proliferating angioblasts in a lesion of subcutaneous angioblastic lymphoid hyperplasia is shown in this field. The cells have an abundant amount of cytoplasm and project into dilated vascular lumens. Some of the cells have cytoplasmic vacuoles, which by their coalescence form lumens in the cords of proliferating endothelial cells.

2. localized in paracortical areas of lymph nodes, in perivascular region of spleen, and in small foci in gastrointestinal tract
3. transformed lymphocyte morphologically characterized by convoluted nucleus (Sezary cell, mycosis cell)

B lymphocytes
1. 20–25% of peripheral blood lymphocytes
2. concentrate in follicular centers of lymph nodes and spleen, and in the lamina propria of the gastrointestinal tract, and intersperse in the bone marrow
3. transformed lymphocyte has plasmacytoid characteristics
4. morphologic expressions that include a small lymphocyte, a cell with a cleaved nucleus, a histiocytoid cells, a stem cell, and a plasmacytoid cell
5. in inflammatory processes, the histologic marker of the B lymphocyte is the plasma cell

In our discussion of lymphocytic dysplasias we emphasized the close relationship between the infiltrating lymphoid cells and the adventitial dermis, particularly the papillary dermis and the perifollicular connective sheath. These forms of lymphocytic dysplasia are characterized by cells with convoluted nuclei (mycosis cells, Sezary cells, Lutzner cells). Evidence has accumulated that the Sezary cell belongs to the T-lymphocyte series. There is increasing evidence that mycosis fungoides and Sezary's syndrome are diseases of the same order, and, by inference, the mycosis cell is also a T lymphocyte. Similar cells with convoluted nuclei have been described in inflammatory processes, particularly lichen planus. We have seen similar cells in the epidermal infiltrates of inflamed seborrheic keratoses. In some examples of lymphomatoid papulosis, lymphoid cells with convoluted nuclei are a significant component of the infiltrates (pityriasis lichenoides, pattern of transformed T-lymphocyte).

If the lymphoid cell with a convoluted nucleus is a marker of reactions and neoplasias of the T-lymphocyte system, then there is histologic evidence that the T lymphocyte is associated with lichenoid changes in squamous epithelium. In particular, lichenoid reactions that are characterized by the migration of lymphoid cells into the epidermal interstitial spaces and by lysis and coagulation of keratinocytes (colloid bodies) appear to be a manifestation of aggressive T lymphocytes.

Reactions involving B lymphocytes, as indicated by the plasma cell as a histologic marker, tend to expand from vascular adventitia but to remain vasocentric. Lupus erythematosus is usually included in general discussions of lichenoid reactions. It is distinguished by a tendency for the dermal infiltrates to remain vasocentric, by relatively limited migration of lymphocytes into the epidermis, and by the presence of plasma cells in the infiltrates. If our concepts are valid, lupus erythematosus may qualify as a lichenoid reaction mediated by B rather than T lymphocytes.

We have illustrated diffuse lymphoid infiltrates at the dermoepidermal junction in a variety of dysplastic and neoplastic processes. Keratinocytic dysplasias are invariably associated with dermal lymphoid infiltrates. In some examples (lichenoid actinic keratoses) the infiltrates partially or completely destroy dysplastic keratinocytes and, in these areas of regression, are associated with lichenoid changes in the surviving keratinocytes. The same sequence of lymphoid infiltrates, focal regression of tumor cells, and lichenoid epidermal patterns may be observed in superficial spreading malignant melanoma. In most of the inflammatory infiltrates that are associated with keratinocytic or melanocytic dysplasias, the reaction has features of both B- and T-cell responses. The infiltrate may migrate into the epidermis to produce lysis of abnormal cells and adjacent normal keratinocytes (T-cell response). The papillary dermal infiltrate commonly contains plasma cells, especially on the reticular dermal side of the infiltrate (B-cell response). In these reactions there may be combined B- and T-cell responses.

The concept of lymphomatoid granulomatosis is of recent origin. Its dermal manifestations are not clearly defined but it is distinguished by its tendency to be vasocentric and vasodestructive. In addition, the infiltrating cells often have plasmacytoid features. Lymphomatoid granulomatosis may be a B-cell response, whereas lymphomatoid papulosa may be a comparable dermal process related to cells of the T-lymphocyte system.

ASSESSMENT OF VARIABLE HISTOLOGIC PATTERNS

On a biopsy specimen the representation of a disease process may not be uniform. Depending on the area selected for examination, diagnostic changes may or may not be present. The spotty nature of the histologic changes may be intrinsic to the process, may be related to the site selected for biopsy by the clinician, may be related to focal involution of the process, or may be related to a technical artifact. If ancillary histologic changes are appreciated, it is sometimes possible to anticipate the need for additional sections or to recommend that the clinician submit additional specimens.

A variety of lesions may show regional variations in patterns that are intrinsic to the process. Superficial spreading basal cell carcinomas may extend in irregular fashions along the basal portion of the epidermis. They may also be multifocal with widely separated nests of cells. Small biopsies of such a specimen may produce poor or inadequate representation of tumor. The apparent multifocality of superficial spreading basal cell carcinoma is in part related to focal areas of spontaneous regression and may be taken as an expression of a defense process by the host.

Lentigo maligna is a lesion characterized by a wide range of histologic patterns. In one or more areas the pattern may be indistinguishable from that of a cellular nevus or a lentigo. If adequate clinical data are supplied on the pathology request form, the need for additional sections from a clinically suspicious, histologically equivocal lentigo maligna may be anticipated. Rarely a melanoma originates in an intradermal nevus. In such a lesion the representation of the nevus cell component may be greater than that of the melanoma. The need for additional sampling of such a lesion may be anticipated if attention is paid to regional variations in patterns, such as focal areas showing nuclear atypism and an increased mitotic rate.

Variability in patterns is less characteristic of the intraepidermal component of superficial spreading malignant melanoma, but is often a feature of the invasive component, particularly that which is confined to the papillary dermis. Commonly nests of melanocytes that are indistinguishable from those of benign nevus cells are present in the dermis in one or more areas in superficial spreading malignant melanomas. Similar nests of nevus-like cells may be in the dermis beneath a lentigo maligna. These cells may be evidence that the melanoma has originated in a preexisting benign nevus, or that the melanoma cells may differentiate, or finally, that melanomas are polyclonal. We favor the interpretation that melanomas are composed of multiple clones (successive generations?) of tumor cells and that some of these are relatively well differentiated and have features similar to those of nevus cells (minimal deviation melanomas).

In some melanomas there are regional variations in pattern that are cytologically atypical but show features of nevus cell differentiation (fasciculation, fibrosis). This is a common feature of acral lentiginous melanomas. In some areas in such a lesion, tumor cells may be loosely arranged in a delicate fibrous matrix. On small biopsy specimens these areas may be confused with those of a benign nevus or interpreted as a variant of blue nevus.

Keratoacanthoma is another tumor in which variation in pattern is a basic feature. This variation is manifested by alternating populations of cytologically benign and cytologically atypical cells. Small superficial biopsies may show only the cytologically benign component. In some instances the atypical component is cytologically malignant and may be indistinguishable from an epidermoid carcinoma.

A second source of difficulty in the interpretation of cutaneous tumors is related to the host's response. Cutaneous carcinomas and melanomas are regularly associated with lymphohistiocytic infiltrates. These infiltrates may be associated with degenerative changes in tumor cells or, in some instances, with partial or complete involution of tumor cells (Fig. 6-78). In keratoacanthomas, involution begins at the deep margin (Fig. 6-79) and progresses by destruction of tumor cells and by fibrosis of the dermis in areas of tumor regression. There is evidence that actinic keratoacanthoma is a polyclonal disease. Involution is accomplished primarily by destruction of abnormal clones with preservation of relatively normal clones, which persist as the epithelial lining of an involuted keratoacanthoma. A regressing keratoacanthoma may show continued active lateral growth in the dermis at a time when involution at the deep margin is well advanced (Fig. 6-80). It would appear that the defense process in the dermis is a local conditioned response. It involves the proliferation of lymphohistiocytic cells and the formation of a reactive stroma. This conditioning response in keratoacanthoma requires approximately 6 weeks for activation and 6 months for full expression. Lateral growth in the dermis is an expression of stromal refractoriness. In actinic keratoacanthomas it may be related to actinically damaged dermal connective tissue. Patterns that resemble keratoacanthoma, particularly the follicular variant, may be

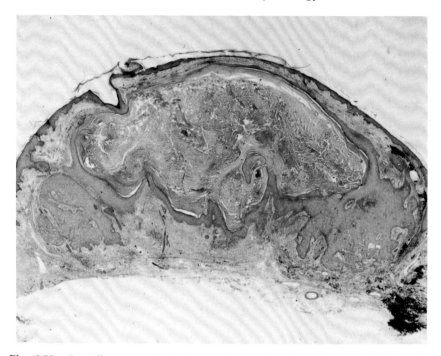

Fig. 6-78. Partially regressed keratoacanthoma showing active growth into the dermis at each lateral margin. The base of the crater is lined by flattened epithelium and shows convincing evdence of regression. The dermis beneath this flattened epithelium is fibrotic and contains infiltrates of chronic inflammatory cells.

seen as a regional variation in basal cell carcinoma and may be a source of error on small biopsies (Fig. 6-81).

The period in which an epithelial tumor actively invades a refractory stroma is basically the histogenetic definition of keratoacanthoma. It might also be spoken of as *acute carcinoma.* When a keratoacanthoma encounters the host's response, it enters a *chronic phase* that is comparable to that of the ordinary forms of cutaneous epidermoid carcinoma. In this phase it is not possible to predict the evolution or involution of individual tumors. Many will completely regress (i.e., they lack the capacity to survive in a conditioned dermis). Focal areas of involution may be present in epidermoid carcinomas (Fig. 6-82).

There are similarities between the host's response to keratoacanthomas and that associated with melanomas. This response is best seen in superficial spreading variants of malignant melanoma. In these lesions the inflammatory process is more or less confined to the papillary dermis. In

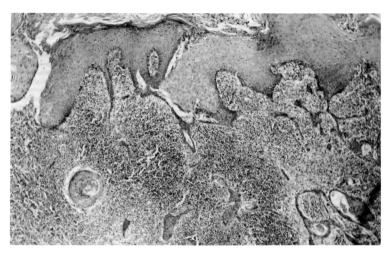

Fig. 6-79. Regressing keratoacanthoma showing thin interconnected cords of cells in inflamed granulation tissue. Clusters of foreign body giant cells and dilated sweat ducts with papillary projections of epithelium in their lumens are present. There is no evidence of a keratinocytic dysplasia in this portion of the lesion. In other areas the lesion showed continued active growth and marked keratinocytic dysplasia.

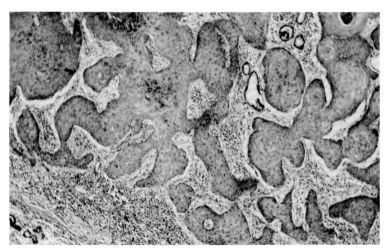

Fig. 6-80. In the same lesion as illustrated in Fig. 6-79 the lateral advancing margin shows continued active growth with no evidence of keratinocytic dysplasia. In this example of keratoacanthoma there is a remarkable regional variation in pattern, ranging from that of a cytologically benign keratoacanthoma to areas that are cytologically indistinguishable from squamous cell carcinoma to areas of partial or complete regression.

143

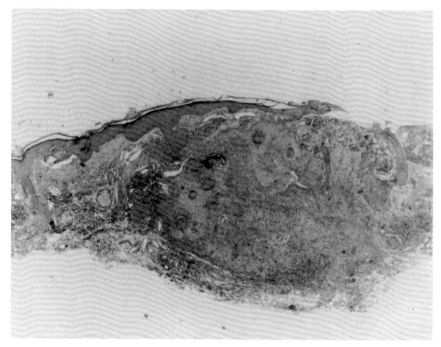

Fig. 6-81. Symptomatic keratoacanthoma at the margin of a basal cell carcinoma. Nests of infiltrating basal cell carcinoma are evident on the right-hand side of the field. The central nodule is composed of hyperplastic keratinocytes that have the cytologic characteristics of those seen in keratoacanthomas. A small biopsy of such a lesion may be misinterpreted as keratoacanthoma.

one or more areas, tumor cells may be completely destroyed. Histologically these appear as "skip-areas" in which the epidermis and papillary dermis are free of tumor. Generally in these areas the epidermis shows hyperkeratosis and effacement of rete ridges. The papillary dermis is thickened and contains tortuous ectatic vessels and spotty infiltrates of lymphocytes and histiocytes. Occasionally the host's response results in complete local involution of the primary tumor. This process is similar to that seen in halo nevi. Cases of this type offer an explanation for the rare examples in which metastatic melanoma is discovered in the absence of a clinically obvious primary tumor.

The focal involution of tumor in these various processes may be a source of error when only small portions of a lesion are available for histologic study (Fig. 6-83). When such material is correlated with clinical diagnoses (e.g., basal cell carcinoma) it is usually possible to anticipate the need for additional sections.

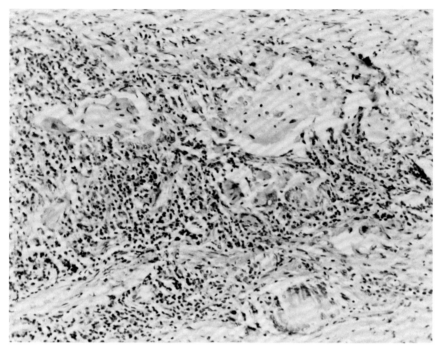

Fig. 6-82. Epidermoid carcinoma showing an area of spontaneous regression. Keratinized degenerating keratinocytes are present in aggregates in an inflamed stroma. Spontaneous regression of tumor is not a distinguishing feature of keratoacanthoma. It may be seen as a regional variation in epidermoid carcinomas.

CONCLUSIONS

Although our presentation of histopathologic problems is diverse, it finds continuity in the repetition of the phenomena of progression and regression in neoplastic systems. These phenomena obviously are not peculiar to experimental neoplastic systems as the bulk of published data over the last two decades would indicate.

A historic example of progression-regression phenomena is provided by Alibert's description of mycosis fungoides. He defined a neoplastic system whose clinical manifestations were those of progression from plaques to tumors over a period of years. If the term mycosis fungoides is to be retained, it should be restricted to those conditions that evolve slowly. Within this neoplastic lymphoid system there may be de novo variants but they are not mycosis fungoides. The quality of progressive step-by-step acquisition of malignant traits is lacking in de novo variants.

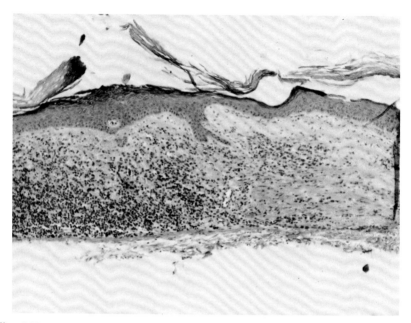

Fig. 6-83. Intermediate keratinocytic dysplasia (carcinoma in situ) showing an area of complete spontaneous regression. The epidermis shows partial effacement of rete ridges. The papillary dermis is thickened and contains a bandlike infiltrate of chronic inflammatory cells. Residual evidence of the keratinocytic dysplasia was present in the epidermis on either side of this area of spontaneous regression.

Progression-regression phenomena are evident in the parapsoriasis-poikiloderma complex. They are obscured by the histologic similarities between reacting and dysplastic lymphoid cells. In the lymphoid system, the regressive phenomena account for the altered vascular and pigmentary patterns that characterize poikiloderma.

Keratoses that are related to actinic exposure may spontaneously regress, may appear in an eruptive fashion following severe exposure, and may progress to carcinomas. The biologic distinction between de novo and actinically induced (evolved) cutaneous epidermoid carcinoma has been clearly defined.

Cellular immune responses are operative in many of the regressive phenomena. At the interface between tumor and normal epithelium, the cellular immune response results in lichenoid patterns. It follows that lichenoid patterns are most often an expression of cellular immunity (T-cell-mediated immunity).

Progressive-regressive phenomena were implicit in Hutchinson's description of lentigo maligna. In the neoplastic melanocytic system they find their clinical expression in variations in color. These variable surface colorations may be used as guides in selecting material for microsectioning. The surface variations in superficial basal cell carcinomas are also expressions of the progressive-regressive phenomena.

At a conceptual level, progressive-regressive phenomena may be influencing the discipline of pathology. We are faced with identity problems. Clinicians want to be pathologists and pathologists want to be financiers. It appears that the discipline of pathology is being fragmented and dismantled. In reality the discipline is intact but diffused. The clinical group that by political design controls the future of dermatopathology has become its instrument. Whether dermatopathology is to progress or regress will be the burden of this instrument.

Bibliography

Arrington, J. H., and Reed, R. J.: Acral lentiginous melanoma. In preparation.

Bauer, W. C., Edwards, D. L., and McGavran, M. H.: A critical analysis of laryngectomy in the treatment of epidermoid carcinoma of the larynx. *Cancer* **15**:263–270, 1962.

Black, M. M., and Wilson Jones, E.: "Lymphomatoid" pityriasis lichenoides; a variant with histological features simulating a lymphoma. *Brit. J. Dermatol.* **86**:329–347, 1972.

Breslow, A.: Thickness, cross-sectional areas, and depth of invasion in the prognosis of cutaneous melanoma. *Ann. Surg.* **172**:902–908, 1970.

Brownstein, M. H., and Helwig, E. B.: The cutaneous amyloidoses: I. Localized forms. *Arch. Dermatol.* **102**:8–19, 1970.

Brownstein, M. H., and Helwig, E. B.: Spread of tumors to the skin. *Arch. Dermatol.* **107**:80–86, 1973.

Caro, W. A., and Helwig, E. B.: Cutaneous lymphoid hyperplasia. *Cancer* **24**:487–502, 1969.

Civatte, J., Laterza, A. M., and Degos, R.: L'hypertrophie des follicules pilosébacés est-elle spéciale a la forme idiopathique de la mucinose folliculaire? *Ann. Dermatol. & Syph.* **99**:47–54, 1972.

Clark, W. C., Jr., Ainsworth, A. M., Bernardino, E. A., Yang, C. H., Mihm, M. C., Jr., and Reed, R. J.: *The Developmental Biology of Primary Human Malignant Melanomas.* Seminars in Oncology, Vol. II, No. 2: 83–103, 1975.

Clark, W. H., Jr., Mihm, M. C., Jr., Reed, R. J., and Ainsworth, A. M.: The lymphocytic infiltrates of the skin. *Human. Pathol.* **5**:25–43, 1974.

Clark, W. H., Reed, R. J., and Mihm, M. C., Jr.: Lupus erythematosus: Histopathology of cutaneous lesions. *Human Pathol.* **4**:157–163, 1973.

Code of Ethics. *Bull. Coll. Amer. Pathologists* **11** (July): 16, 1957.

Copeman, P. W. M., Lewis, M. G., Phillips, T. M., and Elliott, P. G.: Immunological association of the halo naevus with cutaneous malignant melanoma. *Brit. J. Dermatol.* **88**:127–137, 1973.

Daniels, F., Jr.: Ultraviolet carcinogenesis in man, in F. Urbach, (ed.), Conference on The Biology of Cutaneous Cancer, NCI Monograph No. 10, Washington, D.C., pp. 407–422.

Edelson, R. L., Kirkpatrick, C. H., Shevach, E. M., Schein, P. S., Smith, R. W., Green, I., and Lutzner, M.: Preferential cutaneous infiltration by neoplastic thymus-derived lymphocytes: Morphologic and functional studies. *Ann. Int. Med.* **80**:685–692, 1974.

Edelson, R. L., Lutzner, M. A., Kirkpatrick, C. H., Shevach, E. M., and Green, I.: Morphologic and functional properties of the atypical T lymphocytes of the Sezary syndrome. *Mayo Clin. Proc.* **49**:558–566, 1974.

Epstein, E. H., Levin, D. L., Croft, J. D., Jr., and Lutzner, N. A.: Mycosis fungoides —Survival, prognostic features, response to therapy and autopsy findings. *Medicine* **15**:61–72, 1972.

Fisher, H. R.: Ethics in private office practice. *Bull. Coll. Amer. Pathologists* **18** (Jan.): 6–8, 1964.

Flaxman, B. A., Zelasny, G., and Van Scott, E. J.: Non-specificity of characteristic cells in mycosis fungoides. *Arch. Dermatol.* **104**: 141–147, 1972.

Foulds, L.: *Neoplastic Development*, Vol. I., Academic, New York, 1969.

Fraser, J. F.: Mycosis fungoides, its relation to leukemia and lymphosarcoma. *Arch. Dermatol.* **12**: 814–828, 1925.

Fretzin, D. F., and Helwig, E. B.: Atypical fibroxanthoma of the skin: A clinico-pathologic study of 140 cases. *Cancer* **31**: 1541–1552, 1973.

Fuks, Z. Y., Bagshaw, M. A., and Farber, E. M.: Prognostic signs and the management of the mycosis fungoides. *Cancer* **32**: 1385–1395, 1973.

Graham, J. H., Bendl, B. J., and Johnson, W. C.: Solar keratosis with squamous cell carcinoma: A new biologic concept. *Am. J. Pathol.* **55**: 26a, 1969.

Graham, J. H., and Helwig, E. B.: Premalignant cutaneous and mucocutaneous diseases, in J. H. Graham, W. C. Johnson, and E. B. Helwig (Eds.), *Dermal Pathology*, Harper & Row, Hagerstown, Maryland, Chapter 24, pp. 561–624, 1972.

Holdaway, D. R., and Winkelmann, R. K.: Histopathology of Sezary syndrome. Mayo *Clin. Proc.* **49**: 541–547, 1974.

Hudson, A. W., and Winkelmann, R. K.: Atypical fibroxanthoma of the skin: A reappraisal of 19 cases in which the original diagnosis was spindle-cell squamous carcinoma. *Cancer* **29**: 413–422, 1972.

Ive, F. A., Magnus, I. A., Warin, R. P., and Wilson Jones, E.: "Actinic reticuloid": A chronic dermatosis associated with severe photosensitivity and the histological resemblance to lymphoma. *Brit. J. Dermatol.* **81**: 469–485, 1969.

Jeerapaet, P., and Ackerman, A. B.: Histologic patterns of secondary syphilis. *Arch. Dermatol.* **107**: 373–377, 1973.

Johnson, W. C., and Helwig, E. B.: Adenoid squamous cell carcinomas (adeno-acanthoma): A clinicopathologic study of 155 patients. *Cancer* **19**: 1639–1650, 1966.

Kimmelstiel, P.: The modern pathologist. *Arch. Pathol.*: **89**: 193–194, 1970.

Lane, N.: Pseudosarcoma (polypoid sarcoma-like masses) associated with squamous cell carcinoma of the mouth, fauces, and larynx. *Cancer* **10**: 19–41, 1957.

Larson, C. P.: The Kimmelstiel Story. *Bull. Coll. Amer. Pathologists* **12**: 71–72, 1958.

Leavell, U. W., Jr., McNamara, M. J., Muelling, R., Talbert, W. M., Rucker, R. C., and Dalton, A. J.: Orf: Report of 19 human cases with clinical and pathological observations. *J.A.M.A.* **204**: 657–664, 1968.

Lichtiger, B., Mackay, B., and Tessmer, C. F.: Spindle-cell variant of squamous carcinoma. *Cancer* **26**: 1311–1320, 1970.

Liebow, A. A., Carrington, C. R. B., and Friedman, P. J.: Lymphomatoid granulomatosis. *Human Pathol.* **3**: 457–558, 1972.

Lukes, R. J., and Collins, R. D.: Immunologic characterization of human malignant lymphomas. *Cancer* (suppl.) **34**: 1198–1229, 1488–1503, 1974.

Mach, K. W., and Wilgram, G. F.: Characteristic histopothology of cutaneous lymphoplasia (lymphocytoma). *Arch. Dermatol.* **94**: 26–32, 1966.

McGovern, V. J., Mihm, M. C., Jr., Bailly, C., Booth, J. C., Clark, W. H., Cochran, A. J., Hardy, E. G., Hicks, J. D., Levene, A., Lewis, M. G., Little, J. H., and Milton, V. W.: The classification of malignant melanoma and its histologic reporting. *Cancer* **32**: 1446–1457, 1973.

Mihm, M. C., Jr., Clark, W. H., Jr., and From, L.: Current concepts: The clinical diagnosis, classification and histogenetic concepts of the early stages of cutaneous malignant melanoma. *New Eng. J. Med.* **284**: 1078–1082, 1971.

Mihm, M. C., Jr., Fitzpatrick, T. B., Lane Brown, M. M., Raker, J. W., Malt, R. A., and Kaiser, J. S.: Early detection of primary cutaneous malignant melanoma: A color atlas. *New Eng. J. Med.* **289**: 989–996, 1973.

Nagington, J., Tee, G. H., and Smith, J. S.: Milker's nodule virus infection in dorset and their similarity to orf. *Nature* **208**: 505–507, 1965.

Orr, J. W.: The role of the stroma in epidermal carcinogenesis, in Conference on The Biology of Cutaneous Cancer, F. Urbach, (Ed.), NCI Monograph No. 10, Washington, D.C. 531–537.

Pinkus, H.: The borderline between cancer and non-cancer, in A. W. Kopf, and R. Andrade (Eds.): *Year Book of Dermatology*, Year Book Medical Publishers, Chicago, 1967, pp. 5–34.

Pinkus, H.: Anatomy and histology of skin, in J. H. Graham, W. C. Johnson, and E. B. Helwig (Eds.), *Dermal Pathology*, Harper & Row, Hagerstown, Maryland, Chapter 1, pp. 1–24, 1972.

Pinkus, H.: Lichenoid tissue reactions: A speculative review of the clinical spectrum of epidermal basal cell damage with special reference to erythema dyschromicum perstans. *Arch. Dermatol.* **107**: 840–846, 1973.

Pinkus, H., and Mehregan, A. H.: *A Guide to Dermatohistopathology.* Appleton-Century-Crofts, New York, 1969, pp. 102, 400–420, 454–478.

Prehn, R. T.: The immune reaction as a stimulator of tumor growth. *Science* **176**: 170–171, 1972.

Rappaport, H., and Thomas, L. B.: Mycosis fungoides: The pathology of extra-cutaneous involvement. *Cancer* **34**: 1198–1229, 1974.

Reed, R. J.: Atypical fibroxanthomas and spindle-cell carcinomas of the skin. *Bull. Tulane Univ. Med. Fac.* **26**: 75–89, 1967.

Reed, R. J.: Keratoacanthoma: Entity or syndrome. *Bull. Tulane Univ. Med. Fac.* **26**: 117–130, 1967.

Reed, R. J.: Case 17, California Tumor Registry Forty-Seventh Semi-Annual Slide Seminar on Skin and Subcutaneous Tissue, March, 1969.

Reed, R. J.: Actinic keratoacanthoma. *Arch. Dermatol.* **106**: 858–864, 1972.

Reed, R. J.: Primary Cutaneous Reticuloses, PRI Video Digest of Continuing Medical Education, PTH—10, 1972.

Reed, R. J., and Ackerman, A. B.: Pathology of the adventitial dermis: Anatomic observations and biologic speculations. *Human Pathol.* **4**: 207–217, 1973.

Reed, R. J., and Cummings, C. E.: Malignant reticulosis and related conditions of the skin—A reappraisal of mycosis fungoides. *Cancer* **19**: 1231–1247, 1966.

Reed, R. J., Ichinose, H., Clark, W. H., Jr., and Mihm, M. C., Jr.: Common and uncommon melanocytic nevi and borderline melanomas. Seminars in Oncology, Vol. II, No. 2: 119–147, 1975.

Reed, R. J., Meek, T., and Ichinose, H.: Lichen striatus: A histologic model for lichenoid reactions. *Cutaneous Pathol.* **2** (#1): 1–18, 1975.

Reed, R. J., and Terazakis, N.: Subcutaneous angioblastic lymphoid hyperplasia with eosinophilia (Kimura's disease). *Cancer* **29**: 489–497, 1972.

Report of the special ad hoc committee on ethical interpretation. *Bull. Coll. Amer. Pathologists* **22**: 50–51, 1968.

Ryan, E. A., Sanderson, K. V. Barták, P., and Samman, P. D.: Can mycosis fungoides begin in the epidermis? A hypothesis. *Brit. J. Dermatol.* **88**: 419–429, 1973.

Samman, P. D.: The natural history of parapsoriasis en plaques (chronic superficial dermatis) and prereticulotic poikiloderma. *Brit. J. Dermatol.* **87**:405–411, 1972.

Smith, J. L., Jr.: Spindle cell squamous carcinoma, in J. H. Graham, W. C. Johnson, and E. B. Helwig (Eds.), *Dermal Pathology*, Harper & Row, Hagerstown, Maryland, Chapter 26, pp. 631–635, 1972.

Smith, J. L., and Stehlin, J. S.: Spontaneous regression of primary malignant melanoma with regional metastases. *Cancer* **18**:1399–1415, 1965.

Stein, A. A., and Mauro, J.: The future of the practice of pathology. *Bull. Coll. Amer. Pathologists* **24**:53–55, 1970.

Valentino, L. A., and Helwig, E. B.: Lymphomatoid papulosis. *Arch. Pathol.* **96**:409‑416, 1973.

Variakojis, D. Rosas-Uribe, A., and Rappaport, H.: Mycosis fungoides: Pathologic findings in staging laparotomies. *Cancer* **33**:1589–1600, 1974.

Wayte, D. M., and Helwig, E. B.: Halo nevi. *Cancer* **22**:69–90, 1968.

Winkelmann, R. K.: Clinical studies of T-cell erythroderma in the Sezary syndrome. *Mayo Clin. Proc.* **49**:519–525, 1974.

Wise, F.: Parapsoriasis. *NYSJM* **28**:901–908, 1928.

Index